D0190860

Developing a Unified Patient Record

A practical guide

Deb Thompson

EN, RGN, Dip HE

Senior Nurse for Tissue Viability and Practice Development
Weston Area Health NHS Trust, Somerset

and

Kim Wright

RGN, BSc (Hons) Nursing Studies, MSc Health Informatics

Nursing and Midwifery Informatician
North Bristol NHS Trust

Foreword by

Yvonne Baker and Tricia Woodhead

Radcliffe Medical Press

Radcliffe Medical Press
18 Marcham Road
Abingdon
Oxon OX14 1AA
United Kingdom

www.radcliffe-oxford.com
The Radcliffe Medical Press electronic catalogue and online ordering facility.
Direct sales to anywhere in the world.

British Library Cataloguing in Publication Data

A catalogue record for this book is available from the British Library.

ISBN 1 85775 939 7

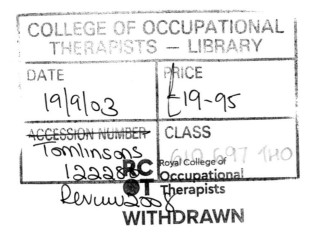
Typeset by Acorn Bookwork, Salisbury, Wiltshire
Printed and bound by TJ International Ltd, Padstow, Cornwall

Contents

Foreword

High quality, shared record keeping is recognised as being fundamentally important to good patient care. There is plenty of evidence about how vital it is, for example in *Learning from Bristol*[1] and *An Organisation with a Memory*,[2] as well as it being a consistent theme in *Information for Health*[3] and all the subsequent strategy documents around health informatics. It is one of the ways we get over the need for professional specialisation whilst taking account of the patient's needs in a holistic manner.

It is very easy to assume that these improvements can only take place when technology is available to support it, but Deb and Kim prove that it is not so much the availability of electronic systems that is key to progress, but cultural change, especially in relation to clinical informatics practice. Quite simply, before technology can help us we need to know what we want to achieve from it. It was this belief that led Weston Area Health NHS Trust and Avon IM&T Consortium to support the New Patient Record project.

This book offers an excellent practical approach to addressing the changes needed in clinical record keeping to support improved patient care, clinical governance, better management information and the move towards electronic patient records (EPRs). It brings together a strong clinical focus with the informatics principles needed to support a successful move to modern record keeping. Using simple tools, Deb and Kim have led the development of a clinical information culture at Weston. These sorts of improvement could be achieved elsewhere as long as there is the will and drive to change.

It is important never to underestimate the challenges of implementing change. This is especially so in clinical practice. Clinical practice is forever changing and healthcare professionals rely on traditional methods of recording patient details to provide consistency. This consistent approach provides an anchor in a challenging world. To change such a fundamental task as record keeping without diminishing patient care takes time, reassurance, education and support. Making sense of change is a key component to successful implementation. Ways of helping staff to make sense of change are fundamental tools of a successful change agent. Deb and Kim provide details of a toolbox and route map to others wishing to take the same progressive step.

This approach is already starting to be adopted locally in other organisations as part of the implementation of electronic records. It has also served as a beacon to other staff groups needing to change their record keeping in preparation for the EPR. From an informatics perspective, we see this work as a vital part of the implementation of electronic records and, ultimately, integrated care records as outlined in *Delivering 21st Century IT Support for the NHS*.[4] We both hope that other communities will be enthused by the practicality and patient focus of what Deb and Kim have done in their hospitals, and feel inspired to do the same.

Yvonne Baker
Divisional Head, Project Management
Avon IM&T Consortium

Tricia Woodhead
Director of Medicine
Weston Area Health NHS Trust

January 2003

References

1   Department of Health (2002) *Learning from Bristol. The Department of Health response to the report of the public inquiry into children's heart surgery at the Bristol Royal Infirmary 1984–1995*. HMSO, London.

2   Department of Health (2002) *An Organisation with a Memory. Report of an expert group on learning from adverse events in the NHS*. HMSO, London.

3   Burns F (1998) *Information for Health. An information strategy for the modern NHS, 1998–2005*. Department of Health Publications, Wetherby.

4   NHS Executive (2002) *Delivering 21st Century IT Support for the NHS*. HMSO, London.

Preface

Kim and I first worked together on a surgical ward in the early 90s and shared common interests in standard setting, documentation and improving patient care. In 1998, Kim led the development of integrated care pathways at Weston. As a junior sister, I first became involved in trustwide record-keeping issues when she became a member of the Stroke Pathway Group. It was through the work of this group that we both developed an insight into the need for a modern framework for collecting clinical information to prepare for electronic patient records.

This inspired the idea for developing a new multidisciplinary system for record keeping, which was facilitated by Kim, and run on the ward that I managed.

I continue to lead clinical record-keeping developments at Weston, whilst Kim has been involved in culture change issues within the Avon IM&T Consortium. The mix of nursing experience and clinical informatics expertise has enabled us to be at the cutting edge of the information agenda in clinical practice.

We wrote this book to help others understand the importance of unified record keeping as an integral part of patient care, and the advantages of designing records in such a way that aggregated clinical information can be easily extracted. Please read and enjoy.

Deb Thompson
Kim Wright
January 2003

About the authors

Deb Thompson EN, RGN, Dip HE is Senior Nurse for Tissue Viability and Practice Development at Weston Area Health NHS Trust in Somerset. She has worked as a nurse within the NHS for 23 years.

Kim Wright RGN, BSc (Hons) Nursing Studies, MSc Health Informatics is a Nursing and Midwifery Informatician at North Bristol NHS Trust. She worked as a ward nurse for 15 years, before spending the last seven years in the NHS in clinical audit, clinical governance and health informatics.

About this book

This practical guide is intended for use by all clinicians and those who deal with clinical information. The book's aims are as follows.

- To put into context the need for a change in the way clinical professionals collect, record, store and use clinical information about patients in acute settings, such as hospitals, with particular reference to the principles within *Information for Health*, the current NHS information strategy.
- To show how clinical governance, including risk management and evidence-based practice, can be more easily addressed by modernising clinical information practice.
- To help those involved in electronic patient record (EPR) procurement to develop a framework for recording care and treatment, which is suitable for transposing to EPR systems.
- To give practical examples of the design and implementation of a unified multidisciplinary patient record.
- To demonstrate how a clinical record can be streamlined to enable management information to be extracted as a by-product of information recorded at the point of care, as part of the care process.

Acknowledgements

We would like to acknowledge the following organisations and people.

The staff and patients of Weston Area Health NHS Trust, Somerset, for their tolerance and participation in the ongoing evolution of record-keeping practice. Particular thanks go to the staff of Birnbeck Ward and the documentation link nurses.

The clinical governance department at Gloucester Royal Infirmary, namely Graham Hodgson and Cheryl Haswell, for allowing us to use and build upon the Gloucester Patient Profile.

Our families, for putting up with our utter distraction from normal life during the writing of this book.

Introduction

History and context

This chapter summarises the evolution of clinical records over the last century, up to the present day, and introduces the concept of change required to modernise record keeping in preparation for an electronic solution.

The written healthcare record has a long history, stemming from the days of Florence Nightingale, and the efforts of doctors to transfer thinking to paper.[1] The creation of the Lloyd-George folder in the 1920s, still in use by GPs, was the start of the recording of medical information. The use of case notes in hospitals started as an *aide-mémoire* for doctors, but has become increasingly complex, multi-dimensional and tied up in bureaucracy.

Within nursing, research shows a tension between the professionalism of using a model of care such as Roper[2] to express nursing work, and the reality of workplace record keeping on the wards.[3] Things have changed since nursing models were introduced, managers now use documentation as a quality assurance mechanism, and all professions are judged by the quality of care. Standards of care are central to the NHS modernisation agenda.[4]

The Audit Commission[5] showed that 25% of clinical time is spent on record keeping, most of which is repetitive. The pressure to document properly to defend against litigation means that records have become little more than an elaborate accounting mechanism.[3] Nurses in particular are being forced to give more attention to record keeping than to nursing care.

Information for Health,[6] the government's strategy to introduce information and information technology (IT) to the NHS, places importance on the need for accurate, concise, person-based information in the context of the electronic patient record (EPR). *The NHS Plan* and *Building the Information Core* merge to give more concrete guidance about how to achieve it. For example:

> *'information systems will need to support health care professionals in addressing the requirements of the earlier modernisation agenda by effective clinical audit information as a by-product of patient care.'*
>
> NHS Executive[4,7]

During the mid 1990s, the Audit Commission looked into the status of hospital and community patient records and drew conclusions about the information within them, the way they were structured, used and stored, and the future.[5,8] One of the main conclusions of the hospital study was that:

> *'before technology can be used effectively, hospitals need to improve their manual systems.'*
>
> *Setting the Records Straight* (p57)[8]

In order for the impact of the impending EPR to be less disruptive, the change in recording to achieve this needs to happen on paper first. We believe that the structure and content of a unified paper record is linked strongly to the successful implementation and use of an EPR.

Assessment is the key to care.[9] The nature of record keeping for each profession is that of individual assessment and free text recording of treatment and care. Unfortunately, each profession undertakes separate assessments, which can be tediously repetitive for the patient/carers. Within comprehensive, unified and timely assessment, routine and repetitive care can be recorded quickly and easily, with attention paid to what is special about the patient, known as 'documentation by exception'.

Integrated care pathways (ICPs) are also central to the modernisation agenda and *Information for Health* – they allow systematic audit, documentation by exception and standardisation of information. In addition, the pathway development process allows all disciplines involved with the patient, from receptionist to clinical coder and clinical professional, to examine processes of care together with the patient at the centre.

In recent years we have recognised that documentation carries a large amount of risk, because of the following.

- Communication between professions is fragmented due to the major differences between the documentation they use. This is compounded by the fact that notes are kept in several different places.
- Nursing care plans are notoriously hard to decipher and because they are time-consuming to complete, the information within them is often of poor quality. Specialist staff often have to duplicate information in two or three different sets of notes to ensure adequate communication.
- In order to follow through an episode of care, for example to answer a complaint, it is necessary to leaf through several different sections of the notes to gain information from the same time period.
- The medical record itself usually includes pages of paper on which is written one sentence, or a page for a risk assessment where the assessment is carried out once during an admission.
- Along with spare sheets filed unnecessarily and an abundance of single fluid charts, the bulk of the notes is increased, contributing to storage and handling problems.

In the late 1990s, the promise of a technological solution to the problems caused by the complexity and inconvenience of paper records was on the horizon. In 1998 the NHS Information Policy Unit (NHSIPU) stated that:

> 'training, cultural changes and improved ways of working are active components in an information-enabled NHS.'
> *Working Together with Health Information*[10]

Clinical practice at the time was focused on ways of working that did not match the working practices needed to make full use of an EPR.

Integrated care pathways

The National Pathways Association[11] describe an integrated care pathway (ICP) as a tool that:

> 'determines locally agreed, multidisciplinary practice based on guidelines and evidence where available, for a specific patient/client group. It forms all or part of the clinical record, documents the care given and facilitates the evaluation of outcomes for continuous monitoring.'
> *Developing Care Pathways*[11]

The development of ICPs has helped to change practice by:

- encouraging a patient-focused, rather than profession-focused, approach to care
- encouraging collaboration between disciplines
- incorporating evidence-based clinical guidelines into everyday practice
- providing a framework for the standardised collection of audit data
- focusing clinical attention on the usefulness of timely, concise and accurate clinical information to aid communication and feed clinical governance returns
- cutting down on less useful free text information, bearing in mind that a future EPR would have difficulty processing free text in a meaningful way
- saving time on record keeping, to free up time for patient care.

Multidisciplinary working tends to be more common due to ICPs, and the work of other services such as the Cancer Collaboration and Booked Admissions. However, although the pathway process is useful in encouraging this change, the resulting *paper* pathway continues to cause problems (*see* Box 1.1).

Box 1.1: Problems with paper ICPs

- Handling patients with multi-disease profiles.
- Filing.
- Recording.
- Training.
- Maintenance and review.
- Tracking and analysis of variances.

The elements of a traditional paper record

Medical notes

Doctors write free text on blank continuation sheets within the case notes, which are generally stored in a trolley at the nurses' station. The medical assessment *process* is systematic; medical assessment leads to the generation of a problem list, which is the basis of any treatment plans. The absence of a written framework means that the medical assessment record can lack consistency. Handwriting is often illegible. Doctors use shorthand for speed and often have separate sections in the case notes, dependent on specialty. This means that, although there is a chronological record, it is often inconsistent, hard to read and in several different places within the case notes. Ongoing patient assessment can be scanty, possibly due to lack of a consistent framework.

Physiotherapy records

Physiotherapists tend to keep separate inpatient notes. The notes are free text and in chronological order, but physiotherapists often write pages of information describing details of treatment and repeat important pieces of information in the medical notes. If the patient continues treatment from home, the record is detached from the case notes and kept in the physiotherapy department. When the patient is discharged from outpatient care the record is filed at the back of the case notes.

Nursing care plans

The Nursing Process was devised by Virginia Henderson in the mid to late 1960s. Nurses translated the principles of Problem, Aim, Action and Evaluate as a way of record keeping as well as a way of nursing. Models of care were created to complement the Nursing Process. Patients were assessed using the Activities of Daily Living.[2] The resulting record was called the nursing care plan and replaced simple free text entry in a record.

This system is still common 25 years later. Care plans are usually kept at the end of the bed, but often collected in at the end of a shift to write in the day's events. This form of nursing practice is such that a full, individualised plan is required for each patient. Audit demonstrates that care plans are often incomplete or missing altogether.[9] There are also many care plans in existence that are handwritten and photocopied to save time, or designed on a home computer and introduced onto individual wards. This can be taken as an indication that the longhand writing out of Problem, Aim, Action and Evaluation is causing too much writing whilst failing to deliver the necessary information and communication function. Furthermore, it demonstrates that certain aspects of care are standard, whatever the patient condition. Common key core care plans are those for hygiene, mobility, pressure area care and so on. An example core care plan is shown in Figure 1.1.

PATIENT CARE PLAN

Date & no.	Patient problem/need		Action
	... is unable to maintain his/her personal hygiene because of ...	1	Maintain privacy by screening bed/bathroom area each time hygiene needs are being attended to.
		2	Assess his/her hygiene needs daily, including hair and teeth. Promote independence within his/her capability.
	Aims ... will state that his/her *own* standards of hygiene have been met daily and he/she feels clean and fresh.	3	Provide him/her with handwashing facilities after using the commode/bottle.
		4	Offer bath/shower where appropriate.
	Care planned by ...	5	Involve his/her relatives/carers in personal care, where appropriate.

CARE GIVEN

Date & no.	Outcome/evaluation	Signed

Figure 1.1 Core care plan for hygiene

Because nurses use a problem-solving approach to care, they record in the same way. This makes care plans many pages long – often two pages per problem. Many ward areas have standard sets of care plans ready to individualise, giving patients up to ten problems caused by admission, and so potentially 20 pages of care plan from day one! The information within the care plans is repetitive and complex and often incomplete. Because of this, the only staff group that uses the information in nursing care plans is nurses. This means that any communication of information to and from other professions has to be written out again in the appropriate place. Specialist staff often record the same information in at least three different sets of records for each patient.

The nursing care plan tends to be filed in the back of the case notes when the patient is discharged, along with other extra documentation, such as charts.

Other professions

Professions such as occupational therapists, speech and language therapists, social workers and visiting doctors often struggle to find the appropriate place to record care and treatment, as many different systems exist within single organisations. Therefore, some also keep their own, more detailed notes. The recent implementation of national risk management standards means that keeping notes separately without indexing the location of each in the main case notes is no longer acceptable.[12]

The record-keeping systems used by the separate professions can work for them, but when viewed from the patient perspective, the following problems emerge.

- The patient is asked the same questions repeatedly to allow separate assessment to take place.
- Communication between professions is difficult, so vital aspects of the patient's illness and hospital stay may be missed.
- Inaccuracies caused by duplication of information may result in problems.
- Physiotherapy and other therapy/specialist notes kept separately from the main case notes may mean that access is easier for outpatient or home visits, but if the patient turns up in A&E, vital aspects of past care and treatment are missing from the information available at the time.

It seems sensible to have a multidisciplinary assessment record for admission that would lead to selection of an ICP. However, experience has shown us that the potential for duplication can be increased by separate assessments that have been built into ICPs to follow national guidelines. Along with the problems listed in Box 1.1 (*see* page 4), it seems that ICPs create *new* recording difficulties. We appreciate that an electronic solution may eventually overcome these difficulties. In the meantime, a generic unified *paper* record can be more versatile than a *paper* ICP by being adaptable according to the needs of the individual.

ICPs continue to be developed, but a unified patient record (UPR) can be the main record of care for every patient. In the UPR, ICPs, or condition-specific mini-plans as an alternative to ICPs, are designed to 'plug in'. They use the same guidelines, layout and terminology as the UPR. In practice, this means that if a patient comes in with a suspected myocardial infarction *and* diabetes, they are assessed using the standard unified assessment. The patient's record is constructed according to individual need and will include recording frameworks and provide guidance for both conditions.

Some may ask 'what is the point of changing from one paper system to another, when EPR is just around the corner?' The answer is that EPR is approaching fast, and work to modernise paper records helps give a practical focus to what is currently a nebulous concept. As professionals start to appreciate the importance of the information they collect, and its use in aggregated form as well as individual patient care, the culture change needed to optimise the use of EPR will follow.

The concept of a unified patient record and the need for a change in culture will be explained in more detail in the next chapter.

References

1   Weed LL (1968) Medical records that guide and teach. *N Eng J Med.* **278**(11): 593–600.
2   Roper N, Logan W and Tierney A (1980) *The Elements of Nursing*. Churchill Livingstone, Edinburgh.
3   Allen D (1998) Record keeping and routine nursing practice – a view from the wards. *J Adv Nurs.* **27**: 1223–30.
4   NHS Executive (2001) *Building the Information Core: implementing The NHS Plan*. NHS Executive, Leeds.
5   Audit Commission (1995) *For Your Information: a study of information management and systems in the acute hospital*. HMSO, London.
6   Burns F (1998) *Information for Health: an information strategy for the modern NHS 1998–2005*. Department of Health Publications, Wetherby.
7   NHS Executive (2000) *The NHS Plan*. Department of Health, London.
8   Audit Commission (1997) *Setting the Records Straight*. HMSO, London.
9   Currell R, Gold G, Hardiker N *et al.* (1998) *The Nursing Information Research Project: final report for the project board*. The NOMINA Group, Leicester.

10   NHS Executive Information Policy Unit (1998) *Working Together with Health Information – a partnership strategy for education, training and development.* Department of Health, London.

11   de Luc K (2001) *Developing Care Pathways: the handbook.* Radcliffe Medical Press, Oxford.

12   NHS Litigation Authority (2002) *Clinical Negligence Scheme for Trusts. Clinical Risk Management Standards.* Wills Ltd, London.

2

What is a unified patient record?

There are numerous ways of describing health records, some of which you will find in the glossary at the back of this book. This chapter introduces the concept of a unified patient record, and uses practical examples from a project undertaken at Weston Area Health NHS Trust in Somerset. There is also discussion about the need for clinical professionals to change their information culture by modernising the way clinical information is collected, stored, analysed and used.

Walsh describes unified case notes as multidisciplinary documentation within a single set of notes, which aims to assess the whole patient in a collaborative way, ensuring that information is realistically documented with clear plans for patient discharge.[1] The notes should ensure that evaluation of care reflects the care the patient has received, highlights changes in care and reasons for those changes, whilst facilitating clinical audit.

This description contains the fundamental elements needed for a unified patient record. Evaluation of the system Walsh described showed a positive impact on the culture of record keeping and multidisciplinary working in the trust where the unified case notes were developed. However, we feel that this concept has the potential to go much further, especially when considered alongside the principles of *Information for Health*[2] (*see* Box 2.1).

> **Box 2.1: *Information for Health* principles**
>
> - Information will be person-based.
> - Systems will be integrated.
> - Management information will be derived from operational systems.
> - Information will be secure and confidential.
> - Information will be shared across the NHS.

For example;

- the 'person-based' ethic can be expanded by giving the patient and carers the opportunity to contribute to the written record
- it is possible to derive management information from clinical assessment recorded at the point of care, as part of care, rather than as a separate exercise
- change of recording framework to the use of documentation by exception allows standardised care to be precisely and quickly recorded, whilst the incorporation of a dynamic evidence base helps to standardise practice.

To encompass the elements above and work towards defining an EPR, it is necessary to design a new way of recording clinical information.

Definition of a unified patient record

We define *our* unified patient record (UPR) as:

> *'A single, collaborative record containing a patient's personal details, diagnosis or condition, assessments, plans, care and treatment. The record system is supported by a dynamic evidence base. The record itself is created and added to by all those who interact with the patient, including the patient. The record fulfils management information needs by using information recorded at the point of care.'*

Multidisciplinary collaboration

Figure 2.1 illustrates the concept of patient-focused care and the multidisciplinary approach.

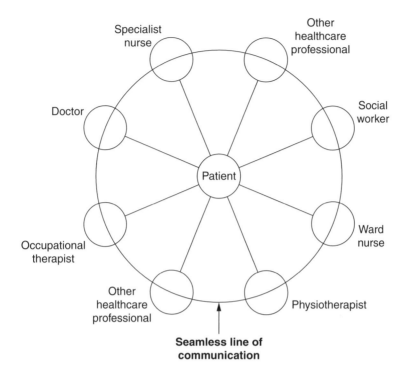

Figure 2.1 A multidisciplinary approach to patient-focused care

In our experience, when a UPR becomes embedded into practice, the circles on the outer wheel diminish to allow the patient to become the focus.

Elements of the unified patient record

This section details the stages of development required for a UPR, illustrated by a project carried out at Weston Area Health NHS Trust. Although the design of each part of any record should be carefully considered, and should be evolutionary, the main focus of the change should be to provide a framework to allow easy collection and use of concise information, shared by all professions.

Collection of demographic data

Professions such as occupational therapists, physiotherapists and social workers traditionally keep separate demographic records, causing unnecessary duplication and repeated requests to the patient for the same information. These professions were involved in the Weston project and collaborated to create a single paper record, easily available to all. The resulting framework for the collection of demographic information is a two-sided document, known as the Front Sheet. The first side holds the patient's demographic details and is based on the former nursing 'Kardex' layout, because the Kardex contained general demographic information and was already useful to all professions. This change in practice has enhanced collaborative working, enabling professions to share and trust each other's information with confidence.

Standardised patient assessment

A framework for assessment should be patient-focused, rather than profession-focused. At Weston, the design of the UPR allows *any* profession to use and share *any* part of the standardised assessment.

The second part of the UPR was originally developed as the Accident and Emergency department (A&E) assessment section of an ICP for stroke. As stroke patients need most A&E diagnostic investigations, the design fits well for all patients, and has reduced duplication. The most significant change to record-keeping practice is the way the document is used. Previously, the A&E nurses started an A&E care plan which was four pages long and often repeated some of the information already in the medical notes, as well as recording some demographic details. When the patient arrived at the ward, the nursing 'Kardex' was commenced, which repeated all of the demographic information, the A&E care plan information and some information from the medical notes. The unified recording framework now starts in A&E and continues on the ward. When it was adopted, four pages of paper were cut out, and unnecessary duplication was stopped.

As the UPR has developed, this piece of the framework seems to have become redundant as an A&E assessment, and has become applicable as a preliminary *general* assessment for all patients. Chapter 5 explains the relevance of this to the local development of EPR and the use of generic functionality rather than a system based on, for example, an A&E module.

The main standardised assessment framework used within the UPR is the Gloucester Patient Profile (GPP). The GPP was created at Gloucester Royal NHS Trust in response to the problem of proliferating patient assessments caused by the introduction of ICPs. The document was designed to:

- provide trend data on patient status and progress
- provide greater objectivity and reliability of patient assessment
- reduce the number of different assessment proformas
- reduce the time taken to complete patient assessment.

It is now used across all the Gloucester Trusts as part of their patient records. The GPP is based on the Barthel assessment, a validated clinical tool for assessing physical function. It allows complete recording of the patient's condition in a format similar to an observation chart. This means that changes in condition can be seen at a glance by whichever profession looks at the chart (*see* Figure 2.2).

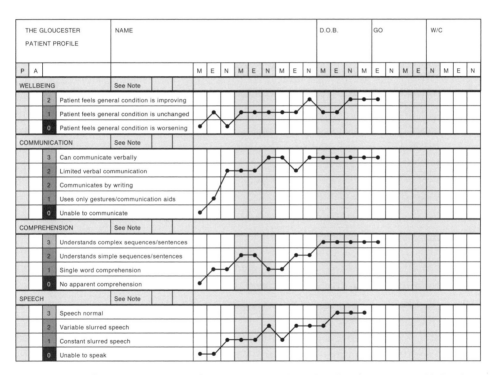

Figure 2.2   Section from the Gloucester Patient Profile (*see* page 89 for key to assessing patient's condition)

The format of the document looks complicated, but once a person becomes familiar with it, it takes less than a minute to complete a single assessment. It reduces the amount of free text needed. It does not, however, replace the need for a record of care; it merely provides a record of the patient's ability and condition to complement it. The GPP works in conjunction with the UPR, particularly the daily/weekly record of care. This means that there is less duplication of recording and that all the essentials of care are included.

The recording framework for the home life assessment originated in the Weston Stroke ICP. The multidisciplinary stroke group worked for three months on the content and layout of the page, to ensure that information and communication needs of all professions were met. Standards for assessment of home circumstances were laid out in the Royal College of Physicians National Guidelines for Stroke[3] – these were incorporated wherever possible.

Assessment for discharge planning created more of a problem. More space was needed to record multidisciplinary home visits, but the stroke group agreed that only a summary would be necessary in the main document. In addition, discharge planning was an ongoing process in stroke rehabilitation, so information was routinely updated in weekly multidisciplinary progress reports. In the same way, this type of progress report can be used for any patient with complex discharge needs. The functionality of an EPR will provide better support for the discharge process, without having the limitations of a paper system. However, the work done to get this far on paper will make a big contribution to the architecture and screen layout of an EPR.

Medical assessment

The medical assessment is based on a standard framework for clerking the patient that has a body systems approach, similar to the traditional medical assessment. However, the home life assessment has already been recorded and is shared within the UPR, so the doctor has no need to duplicate the information. The assessment concludes with a problem list and action points that are updated at set points during the stay and at discharge. This facility adds clarity to the patient's plan and also helps when constructing a discharge summary.

Planning and recording care

Unified condition-specific mini-plans can be presented in table format and are similar to a task list, following the format of a 5-day plan (see Figure 2.3). There are sections for clinical care, guidelines for activity and other care and each can forward plan tasks for the patient. Care within the 5-day plan can be predicted and pre-recorded, or prescribed individually according to need. Standardised care is predicted according to guidelines for certain conditions. An example of non-standardised care might be if a patient falls out of bed and requires a check X-ray the next day. This will be recorded on the 5-day plan and signed off by a member of the team when completed. This page is useful as a quick summary of patient care, and for reference when looking at tests and investigations that have been completed.

Date commenced:

Write additional notes/variations from the plan on the

multidisciplinary variations page

Hospital no:

Name:

DoB:

(affix label)

*if indicated

Please note – you do not need to initial everything every day. These are reminders of the issues that should be considered.

	Day 1 Admission	Sig	Day 2	Sig	Day 3	Sig	Day 4	Sig	Day 5	Sig
Secondary prevention	ECG 1 Cardiac enzymes 1 Consider TEDS* ACE Statin		ECG 2 Cardiac enzymes 2		ECG 3 Cardiac enzymes 3 ? ETT					
Guidelines of activity	Bed rest Refer to cardiac rehab nurse		Sit in chair – am (1/2 hour) Walk one way to the toilet – pm		Walk both ways to the toilet Sit out in chair for longer periods		Walk around the ward Pre discharge rehab advice		Bath/shower Consider discharge	
Other care	Weight Waterlow Cannula check Pain assess		Cannula check Pain assess Psychological support		Cannula check – remove/replace Pain assess Plan discharge		Pain assess Waterlow		Pain assess	

Figure 2.3 Example of a 5-day plan

Medical protocols and unified condition-specific mini-plans have been developed that plug into the UPR. For instance, the acute cardiac chest pain protocol can be utilised for any patient with chest pain. This can be activated at any time during their stay, rather than needing to commence an ICP as well as the current record. The format described in this section is very much in keeping with the most favourable architecture of an EPR.[4]

Essentials of care

Once the initial patient assessment has been completed using the GPP, a plan can be designed according to the needs of the individual. All patients have essential requirements of care, including:

- hygiene
- pressure area care
- mobility
- intake
- communication
- discharge.

Therefore, when designing a document to record care, headings can be standardised to *predict* care needs. Statements about care are given as outcomes, for example, 'patient is free from sore areas'. This means that the clinician initials to say it is so. If the statement is not true, the clinician must use the variation page to give a reason and record action taken. To *individualise* the plan, care guides and complex care plans needed for this patient are recorded on this page, and staff sign to confirm when the care has been delivered.

Recording of the essentials of care can be presented in several different formats based on the acuity of patient needs – this can be daily, weekly or, less commonly, hourly. The framework is designed to allow quick and easy recording of everyday care.

Daily record of care

This is two-sided and each side can hold two days of care. Each daily section is the same and is structured in a similar way to the GPP in that there is room to record three times a day, morning, evening and night (MEN).

DAILY RECORD OF CARE

Ward:

Date:

Hospital no:
Name:
DoB: Affix label here

Please initial appropriate box as each item is considered and action completed

Guidelines to be followed/care to be given	M	E	N		M	E	N
Assistance with hygiene (see GPP)				**Patient/carer communication**			
Patient has had: bath/shower/assisted wash/shave				Psychological wellbeing			
mouthcare/hair washed				Patient feels supported and well-informed			
				Relatives have been included			
Pressure area care							
Patient is free from sore areas				**Discharge**			
Preventative plan has changed (Y/N)				Review ongoing care needs			
				Action towards discharge taken			
Mobility							
Last assessment followed				**Complex care plans used today** (please list)			
Assessment modified as required							
Complex care plan in use? (Y/N)							
Intake				**Care guides used today** (please list)			
Cannula in situ Y/N							
Phlebitis score is 0							
Cannula last changed on:							
Intake is acceptable							
All meals have been eaten							

Figure 2.4 Section from the daily record of care

Weekly record of care

Although the view is different, the standard headings are the same as those in the daily record. This allows a week's care to be recorded on one page for those patients who are chronically ill and whose care needs do not change on a daily basis. The weekly record of care is mostly used for medical patients.

WEEKLY RECORD OF CARE

Week commencing:	M	E	N	M	E	N	M	E	N	M	E	N	M	E	N	M	E	N	M	E	N
Assistance with hygiene (see GPP)																					
Bath/shower/hair washed																					
Assisted wash																					
Mouthcare																					
Shave																					
Pressure area care																					
Patient is free from sore areas																					
Care guide in use (Y/N)																					
Mobility																					
Last assessment followed																					
Complex care plan in use? (Y/N)																					
Intake																					
No. of cannulae in situ																					
Cannula 1 phlebitis score is 0																					
changed today																					
record site daily																					
Cannula 2 phlebitis score is 0																					
changed today																					
record site daily																					
Intake is acceptable																					
All meals have been eaten																					

Figure 2.5   Section from the weekly record of care

Hourly record of care

This is designed to reflect the needs of acutely ill patients, such as those in intensive or high dependency care. The structure of the record is the same in that headings are used for sections, but the headings are different. They are based on body systems to conform to critical care models.

HOURLY RECORD OF CARE

Date:	Time											
Respiratory system (see GPP)												
Hourly observations carried out												
Patient is breathing spontaneously												
F1O2 > 50%												
CPAP												
BIPAP												
IPPV												
ETT												
Tracheostomy present?												
ETT or tracheostomy suction performed												
Respiratory arrest?												
Cardiovascular system												
Hourly observations carried out												
Cardiac monitoring												
Inatropes												
Arterial line in use (see care guide)												
CVP line in situ												
CVP measurements taken												
IV access – no. of cannulae												

Figure 2.6 Section from the hourly record of care

Complex care plan

This part of the record was designed to allow planning of elements of care that were not predicted in the record of care or included in the care guides (full explanation of their purpose is on page 35). For example, if a patient has a complex wound, with an unusual dressing regime, it is impossible to devise a care guide as the approach to care needs to be individualised. Therefore, the person assessing the patient writes guidelines on the complex care plan. These guidelines are based on clinical knowledge and supported by general policies and protocols. Adherence to the plan is recorded on the daily or weekly record. The complex care plan was in frequent use at the start of the project but, as the number of evidence-based care guides has increased, the need for complex care plans has declined. Further evolution of this concept has occurred with the development of specialist records. For example, the tissue viability record provides a sub-framework for detailed wound management information, replacing the need for free text complex care (*see* page 26).

Variation record

The variation record is the place where all professions record important information that differs from everyday care. Care can be recorded on a unified page using free text. The profession is identified by the use of a code in the left hand column. If a sudden change in condition occurs, or treatment changes, writing it on the variation record will ensure that all professions see it. Routine nursing care is consigned to the daily or weekly record but variations to the care are recorded. This is known as 'recording by exception'. An example of this might be if a nurse is unable

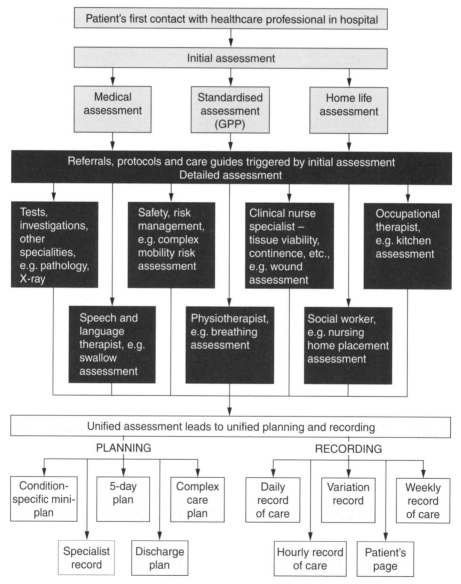

Figure 2.7 Process of assessment, planning and recording within a UPR

to sign to say 'oral intake is acceptable'. He or she may record this on the variation record, along with action taken, e.g. 'doctor informed and patient now being given hourly fluids'.

In the UPR model we have described, the record can be expanded to encompass all complexities within healthcare, whilst maintaining the core principles of *Information for Health*, detailed in Chapter 1. Figure 2.7 clearly demonstrates how unified generic assessment can start the process of patient care in hospital and allow drilling down from standard record to specialist record. An EPR might use this type of architecture.

How does this work in practice?

This section gives an example of how a generalised assessment can lead to a detailed assessment. Audit of the mobility risk assessment in the former nursing documentation found that it was usually carried out once on admission. If a patient was at risk, a nursing care plan was commenced. However, the plan was rarely updated, and re-assessment never took place. The importance of re-assessment is in the subsequent moving and handling needs of both patient and staff. Physiotherapists, occupational therapists and nurses worked together to find a way of incorporating a quick but useful daily assessment of mobility, combined with a more detailed assessment and record for those needing manual help. It was decided that, by putting the daily risk assessment on the GPP, it would be carried out along with the other assessments. The trend layout of the GPP allows easy comparison with previous assessments. The GPP asks the question 'is the complex assessment up to date?' and requires a daily yes/no answer (*see* Figure 2.8).

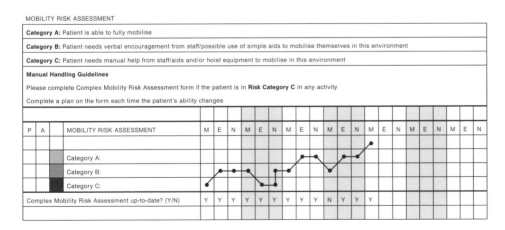

Figure 2.8 Mobility risk assessment section from the GPP (*see* page 89 for key to assessing patient's condition)

The risk assessment is colour-coded 'red, yellow and green' for ease of use. This means that, if a patient drops to 'red' in an activity, a complex mobility assessment and plan need to be commenced and updated when ability changes. The complex assessment is designed to allow the recording of sets of chronological information to form a record based around safe systems for moving and handling (*see* Figure 2.9).

The information is recorded on one page and includes:

- the date of the latest complex assessment
- the signature of the assessor
- the type of movement needed, e.g. lying to sitting – called 'the task'
- the equipment and number of people needed to perform the task.

The page is double-sided and allows for seven re-assessments before a new sheet is needed.

COMPLEX MOBILITY RISK ASSESSMENT

This patient's mobility has been assessed for risk and should therefore mobilise as shown below.

Name: Unit no:

	Date with signature and recommended equipment			
Task				
Turn to right in bed				
Turn to left in bed				
Up and down bed				

Figure 2.9   Section from the complex mobility risk assessment page

Although this process appears complex, it works well in practice, as illustrated by the model in Figure 2.7.

Specialist records

As explained, general patient assessments can lead onto specialist assessments. This is where the record has the ability to expand according to the patient's needs. With this function, specialist information can be recorded in a standardised way. An example of this is where the patient has been assessed on the GPP as having a pressure ulcer. Previously, the nurse would develop a complex care plan detailing the care required for this patient's wound and list that the pressure ulcer prevention care guide was being used to provide guidelines for staff that would prevent further pressure damage occurring. This method seemed reasonable, as originally it was felt that the approach to wound care could not be standardised due to the individual complex patient needs involved. However, the process was lengthy and open to error, as the content of the complex care plan for the wound depended on the level of nurse knowledge and often important information was missed. For example, in wound care it is important to record the grade, size, site and condition of the wound on initial assessments and each time the dressing is changed.[5] In an acute environment, continuity of care can be compromised by the number of different healthcare professionals involved in management of the wound. Therefore, the information recorded should provide each healthcare professional with a mental picture of the wound. By recording the information in a standardised way each time the wound is assessed, progress can be easily monitored by looking at the trends the record provides. This allows staff to evaluate the effectiveness of the care the patient is receiving. Initially, within the UPR, information regarding wound care was recorded on the variation record. This approach resulted in poor quality, fragmented information that was difficult to locate within the free text. Therefore a tissue viability record was designed (*see* Figure 2.10). This is a multi-functional record on one double-sided piece of A4 paper. It has been designed in such a way that information about pressure ulcers is collected at the point of care but, on discharge, the information is transferred into a pressure sores database (for full explanation *see* Chapter 5). Previously, the recording of a pressure ulcer assessment could take up to 45 minutes. With the implementation of the tissue viability record this has been reduced to ten minutes. The information contained within the record is far more concise and provides good quality data.

Classification of wound (please tick the appropriate box)	Other disciplines involved (please specify)
☐ Surgical ☐ Traumatic ☐ Leg ulcer ☐ Foot ulcer ☐ Cellulitis ☐ Pressure sore (If pressure sore complete next section)	☐ Dietitian ☐ Orthopaedic surgeon ☐ Vascular surgeon ☐ Plastic surgeon

Pressure sore details
Grade (1–5 Torrance scale – please specify)   Damage on admission ☐ Yes ☐ No
Waterlow score? (please specify)   Referred to tissue viability nurse ☐

Relevant history of pressure sore or contributing factors

Equipment in use
☐ Pressure reducing foam mattress   ☐ Alternating pressure mattress
☐ Pressure relieving cushion   ☐ Leg troughs and bed cradle
☐ Pressure relieving chair   ☐ Other (please specify)

Figure 2.10   Section from the tissue viability record

The process of drilling down levels of assessment, planning and recording seems complex but it achieves the following.

- Condensing of assessment and ongoing evaluation, for example, of a wound.
- Specification of a framework for collecting good quality information.
- Provision of a structure for staff to follow, with less paper.
- Reduction in the time spent recording information.
- Provision of quality information for audit and educational purposes.
- Compliance with Health and Safety Regulations for Moving and Handling Patients, and providing a record of this.
- Condensing of multidisciplinary assessment and planning from separate records into one record.
- Easier and more concise recording of information.
- The use of multidisciplinary expertise in the development and implementation of guidelines, for example, the mobility risk assessment.

Patient involvement

Patient involvement is high on all NHS agendas.[6] Participation in care is seen as key to informed decision making and patient satisfaction, as well as being key to restoring the public's faith in the NHS. Patients are involved in this model of unified record in the following ways.

Self-assessment

Regular assessment via the GPP begins with patient self-assessment. This helps to improve communication and reassure both staff and patient that they are going in the same direction (*see* Figure 2.11).

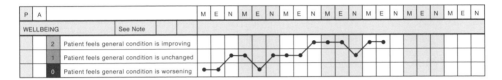

Figure 2.11 Patient self-assessment section of GPP

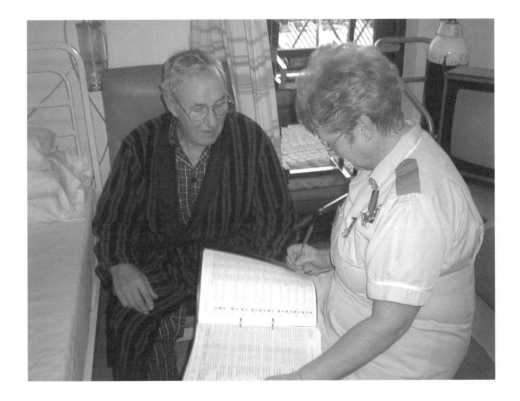

Figure 2.12 Staff and patients complete the GPP together

Patients value being asked, and often take the opportunity to voice other concerns which may previously have been left undetected. Anecdotal evidence suggests that intervention at this early stage prevents complaints.

Contributing to the record

The patient's page is a key part of the record (*see* Figures 2.12 and 2.13). It allows patients and carers the opportunity to contribute to the written record and is designed to ensure that the patient can have influence over their care. When a patient is admitted, the nurse explains that the patient can look at their record and make comments about their care. If they cannot find someone when they need to say something or ask questions, they can write on the patient's page, and their query will be answered as soon as possible.

PATIENT'S PAGE

Ward:
Date:

	Hospital no:
Name:	
DoB:	Affix label here

This page is for you to record any comments, or to raise concerns you may have about aspects of your care and the service we provide. Your relatives/carers are also welcome to write on this page. Your care will not be prejudiced by what you write here. You might like to write about:

- any concerns or comments about your treatment or hospital stay
- any questions you would like answered
- any concerns about your discharge from hospital.

Date	Comments

Figure 2.13 Section from the patient's page

The page is filed as part of the record, whether the patient has used it or not. The idea for the page came about from a patient satisfaction survey, where the issue brought up most was lack of information for patients. It was part of a series of improvements, including:

- information cards for relatives with the ward sister's and consultants' names and phone numbers

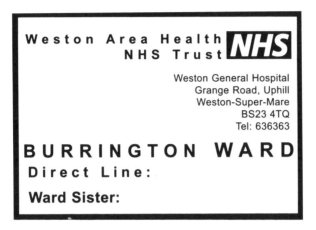

Figure 2.14 Information card

- taping of consultations with medical staff, for later playing back to relatives and carers
- provision of bedside tape players.

The patient's page and information cards were commended as good practice at a recent Commission for Health Improvement (CHI) visit.[7] When comments have been written on the patient's page, responses have been effective in giving patients the information they want, and for stopping potential complaints.

Benefits of a unified patient record

Benefits for patients and carers

By using a UPR patients can receive better care through:

- better collaboration and communication between disciplines
- reduced need for the patient and carers to provide the same information repeatedly
- less duplication of recording, freeing up time from record keeping for professionals to spend on patient care
- ensuring the patient receives the same standard of care wherever they are
- ensuring that the patient gets up-to-date care and treatment, based on best evidence
- giving the patient the opportunity to contribute to the record in a way that is meaningful for them.

Benefits for staff

Staff can achieve the following benefits by using a UPR.

- A patient-focused, rather than profession-focused, approach to care.
- The opportunity to appraise evidence and create care guides, increasing confidence and motivation when delivering care.
- Allows staff to focus on real issues, and provides a framework with an end point that is applied to practice, rather than being a paper exercise.
- The integration of evidence-based clinical guidelines into the UPR, ensuring behaviour-change in the delivery of care, rather than just increasing knowledge.
- Better representation of trends in the patient's condition using the GPP, allowing staff to monitor the patient's condition more effectively.
- All professions have easy access to each other's care record, allowing the patient to be seen as a whole, rather than in separate pieces.
- Less writing and less duplication of information.
- Clinical attention is focused on the usefulness of timely, concise and accurate clinical information to aid communication and feed clinical governance returns.
- Doctors use the GPP as a summary of the patient's condition – deterioration and improvement in condition can be spotted at a glance.
- Referral to other services/external agencies can be made objectively using the functional assessment score on the GPP.

- Time is saved because A&E staff assess on the same record – time-consuming separate initial assessment on the ward is no longer necessary.
- Because information is more precise and better organised, communication between professions is improved.
- Less time is spent waiting for verbal confirmation of condition – saves on ward round time.
- Records of care focus on what is special about the patient, rather than documenting routine care, day after day.
- The record is standard across the organisation, making it easier for staff to access information and use the record, whichever clinical area they are in.

Benefits for the organisation

The use of a UPR within the organisation provides the following benefits.

- Ongoing contribution to the body of knowledgeable and informed practitioners.
- Provides a framework for the standardised collection of clinical audit data.
- Cuts down on the use of less important free text information, bearing in mind that a future EPR would have difficulty processing free text in a meaningful way.
- Allows filing of care and treatment in chronological order, rather than separate professions' sections in the case notes, thus allowing the patient's progress to be followed with ease.
- Less paper is generated, meaning lessened storage and handling problems.
- The record-keeping system is updated to ensure integrated, streamlined and standardised records, ready for EPR.
- Lowers the risk of litigation through more complete record keeping, evidence-based care, easier answering of complaints and increased patient satisfaction.
- Helps preparation for Clinical Negligence Scheme for Trusts (CNST) assessment by creating truly unified records and patient-focused care.
- Automatic monitoring of pressure sore information, as clinical governance assistants routinely input the information from the GPP, and reports can be generated from the Patient Administration System (PAS). This same model could potentially be used to collect and process other clinical information for clinical governance purposes.

- There is potential for using the GPP as a standardised dependency scoring system. This information could be collected as part of assessment (colour-based – *see* the GPP) rather than a separate, tedious and time-consuming paper exercise.

Finally ...

The Weston record-keeping project has changed record-keeping practice, but has also had an impact on quality of care, with a way of ensuring that evidence-based guidelines are actually used in practice. Within an ever-changing NHS that has rising consumer demands, it seems that a UPR is a sensible solution to improving care and protecting clinicians in their everyday work. Documentation by exception is minimalist in its approach, and, as such, requires an evidence-based foundation. Without this, healthcare professionals' accountability is open to question. The next chapter goes into more detail about evidence-based practice, and the opportunity the UPR provides to bridge the theory–practice gap.

References

1   Walsh C (1998) Patient records improve with unified case notes. *Nursing Times*. **94**(24): 52–3.
2   Burns F (1998) *Information for Health: an information strategy for the modern NHS 1998–2005*. Department of Health Publications, Wetherby.
3   Royal College of Physicians (1999) *National Guidelines for Stroke*. RCGP, London.
4   van Bemmel JH and Musen MA (1997) *Handbook of Medical Informatics*. Springer-Verlag, Heidelberg.
5   European Pressure Ulcer Advisory Panel (2001) *Pressure Ulcer Treatment Guidelines*. EPUAP Business Office, Oxford.
6   NHS Executive (2000) *The NHS Plan*. Department of Health, London.
7   Commission for Health Improvement (2001) *Report of a Clinical Governance Review at Weston Area Health NHS Trust*. The Stationery Office, London.

3

The use of evidence-based practice within a unified patient record

This chapter will describe the origins and importance of evidence-based medicine (EBM), its relationship to evidence-based practice (EBP) and its relevance in the development of what are known as care guides, an integral part of the UPR.

Evidence-based practice

The origins of EBM in the UK can be traced back to Archie Cochrane.[1] Cochrane's first publication was in 1972 and entitled *Effectiveness and Efficiency: random reflections on the health service.* The Cochrane centre was founded in 1992 as part of the NHS Research and Development programme; this led to the development of the Cochrane Collaboration. The Cochrane Collaboration is now a worldwide resource that maintains and disseminates research findings. In the mid 90s, David Sackett established the UK centre for EBM in Oxford. This centre is now a key focus for disseminating teaching and evaluating EBM throughout the UK, and is linked to the Cochrane Collaboration.[2] The newly available National Electronic Library for Health (www.nelh.nhs.uk) gives wider access to all forms of evidence via NHSnet:

> 'an authoritative source of current healthcare knowledge to improve clinical practice and enable the most appropriate treatment to be provided based on accredited clinical evidence.'
>
> Building the Information Core[3]

The growth of consumerism and legislation through government policy have driven EBP firmly to the top of the NHS agenda.[4,5]

- Consumerism – people are more aware about personal health issues. Information about health and illness is more freely available via media and the Internet.[4]
- Legislation – the push to modernise the NHS has put the patient at the forefront of decision making about health. The emphasis is on the knowledge management by professionals and decision-making partnerships with the patient.[6]

The government has recognised that there is a need to restore the public's faith in the NHS and the quality of service it provides. To enable this change a clinical governance framework has been designed to assist healthcare professionals to improve and maintain quality of care. A mainstay of this strategy is EBP, research and development (R&D) and continuing professional development (CPD).[7,8]

Muir Gray[6] who worked with David Sackett at the Oxford centre defines EBP as:

> 'an approach to decision making in which the clinician uses the best evidence available, in consultation with the patient, to decide which option suits the patient best.'
>
> Evidence-based Healthcare[6]

The EBM approach to research findings can be a valuable tool for clinical decision making. It is often the translation from theory into practice that proves difficult. The introduction of care guides as part of a UPR can help to bridge the theory–practice gap.

The key to the practical application of EBP is to remain focused on the patient and for each clinician to take responsibility for his or her decisions. Within these decisions, the clinician must be confident that he or she is delivering the best possible care for the individual patient. EBP should be the application of research along with clinical expertise and the patients' preferences.[9]

Care guides

In the Roper model of care, adopted by British nurses as a way of recording, care actions are made explicit by writing them out in full in the record in the form of a care plan. This has given nurses the security of thinking that, because an explicit individualised care plan exists, it will support them in their professional accountability. However, care plans may exist, but they are not evaluated regularly.[10] This means that a record of *care given* does not exist.

As previously mentioned, the UPR uses documentation by exception as a way of reducing writing and paper, whilst maintaining a complete record of care. Documentation by exception needs to be supported by a dynamic evidence-base – this is provided by care guides. Care guides are simply guidelines detailing aspects of everyday care. They are created from evidence, as illustrated in Figure 3.1, and exist to provide an agreed standard of care across the organisation. They should complement but never replace the judgement of the clinician, who has knowledge of both the patient and the evidence.

The model by Bury and Mead[11] has been adapted in Figure 3.1 to illustrate how care guides can fit into the evidence-based practice.

If the care guide in Figure 3.2 is compared to the core care plan in Chapter 1 it can be seen that the two are similar.

During the development and piloting of the UPR at Weston, groups of nurses on the pilot ward took an aspect of care previously detailed on a care plan and reviewed the evidence related to it. The resulting evidence-based guidelines acted as support for nurses in the carrying out and recording of care. The guidelines were put into folders and placed in ward areas, so that nurses could refer to them as and when they needed to.

By the time the UPR was ready to be rolled out, the guidelines had evolved into care guides, a term which it was felt better described their intended use. Qualitative evaluation of the UPR has shown that the most useful part of the system is the care guides.

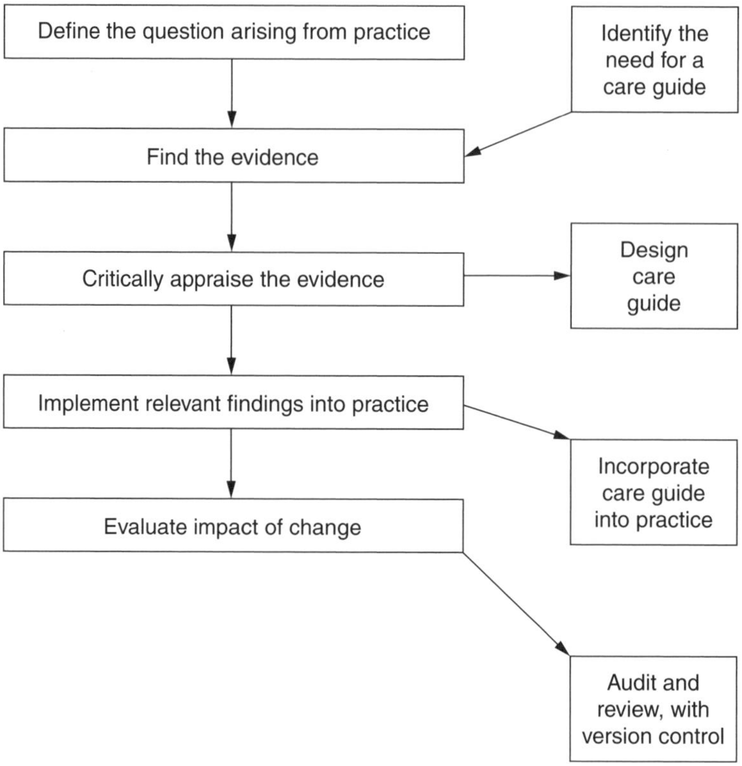

Figure 3.1 Care guide development applied to the Bury and Mead
EBP model

Bank/agency and new staff find the care guides particularly useful. It is
the responsibility of the clinician to make him or herself aware of the care
guide(s). If someone signs to say they have followed a care guide(s), but do
not know its content, they could be open to litigation. For this reason, it is
important to maintain a history of each care guide, via version control.

The report of the recent CHI visit to Weston stated about the care
guides:

> 'the trust has a good foundation for continuing work on guidelines and
> integrated care pathways.'
>
> *Clinical Governance Review*[12]

It also recommended a central register, available to all staff. In order to
ease access to the care guides, they have been converted to read-only
documents and put on the trust intranet. This has been progressed to
coincide with the launch of the intranet to all clinical staff, and also

---

Care Guide for Hygiene Needs

1 Each patient should be offered daily hygiene facilities appropriate to their needs. For details of procedures such as bed-bathing and general mouth care, refer to the Royal Marsden Manual of Clinical Procedures. Independence to be maintained wherever possible, and assistance given where needed.

2 For patients who are unable to indicate their wishes, full hygiene care should be given.

3 Maintain privacy by screening bed/bathroom area each time hygiene needs are being attended to.

4 Ensure that toilet needs are attended to whenever necessary, and that the call bell is within reach for patients who need assistance.

5 Offer the patient hand-washing facilities each time he/she uses the commode/urinal.

6 Involve relatives/carers as appropriate.

Author:
Date of approval: November 2000
Date of last review: July 2001
Date of next review: July 2002
Version 1.0

Figure 3.2 Hygiene care guide

means that staff will see familiar information when they access it. The longer-term plan involves the creation of a searchable database containing *all* guidelines. Key words have been identified from each of the care guides, in order to create the database.

For patients, the main benefit of care guides is that they receive evidence-based care to the same standard wherever they are in the trust. This differs from the traditional approach, where care is often based on custom and practice, as well as anecdotal evidence.

There are many guidelines available to inform practice. However, in our experience, the involvement of groups of staff in the research and production of local care guides provides far more benefit in terms of ownership and commitment to using them within the UPR. Also, staff are keenly aware of the need for regular review and updating of practice via the care guides.

Finally ...

This chapter has focused on the need to base practice on evidence, and the use of care guides as a practical tool to enable this to happen. The process of building care guides has been valuable, both for current clinical practice, and for building the knowledge base. In future EPR will ensure that this type of evidence base is at the clinicians' fingertips. The next chapter details the links between paper and electronic records.

References

1   Cochrane A (1972) *Effectiveness and Efficiency: random reflections on the health service*. The Cochrane Library, Issue 4. Update Software, Oxford.
2   Sackett DL, Strauss SE, Richardson SW *et al*. (2000) *Evidence-based Medicine. How to Practice and Teach EBM*. Churchill Livingstone, London.
3   Department of Health (2001) *Building the Information Core – implementing The NHS Plan*. HMSO, London.
4   Grayson L (1997) *Evidence-based Medicine*. The British Library Board, London.
5   Salvage J (1998) Evidence-based practice: a mixture of motives? *NT Research*. **1**(6): 419–20.
6   Gray JAM (1997) *Evidence-based Healthcare*. Churchill Livingstone, Edinburgh.
7   Department of Health (1997) *The New NHS: modern and dependable*. HMSO, London.

8   Department of Health (1997) *A First Class Service: quality in the new NHS.* HMSO, London.

9   DiCenso A and Cullum N (1998) Implementing evidence-based nursing: some misconceptions. *Evid Based Nurs.* **1**(2): 38–40.

10 Hotchkiss R (1997) Integrated care pathways. *NT Research.* **2**(1): 30–6.

11 Bury JT and Mead MJ (1998) *Evidence-based Healthcare: a practical guide for therapists.* Butterworth Heinemann, Oxford.

12 Commission for Health Improvement (2001) *Report of a Clinical Governance Review at Weston Area Health NHS Trust.* The Stationery Office, London.

4

The link between record keeping and an EPR

This chapter focuses on clinical record keeping and the concept of EPR, and the ways in which they are inextricably linked, including:

- the capacity of each method to support patient-focused care
- the pros and cons of clinical language within records
- the importance of structured information
- a way of ensuring modernisation of paper systems is carried through to electronic systems.

The standard definition of an electronic patient record (EPR) is:

'a record containing a patient's personal details (name, date of birth, etc.), their diagnosis or condition, and details about the treatment/assessments undertaken by a clinician. Typically covers the episodic care provided mainly by one institution.'

Information for Health[1]

In fact, the EPR has the potential to be much more than the definition, by virtue of the functionality listed in the EPR levels discussed later in the chapter.

The UPR, as described in Chapter 2, makes great improvements over traditional records when it comes to patient focused-care. However, in theory, the EPR has the advanced functionality needed to improve the patient experience by:

- streamlining processes such as booking appointments and being referred to specialist services
- enabling better communication between professions and support services, such as laboratories
- making easier access and use of evidence to support practice
- 24 hour a day instant access to any record, wherever it is needed
- speeding up of communication between acute and primary, meaning that the patient gets more timely diagnosis and treatment
- automation of background services such as ordering drugs, managing beds and theatre time
- improved risk management by use of alerts.

This is not an exhaustive list, but is dependent upon the level of implementation and usage of the EPR.

Clinical language issues

In order for patient records to support healthcare team working, the language they use must be common to all professions. At present, classification systems are used to apply standard coding to written clinical information. In theory, this allows consistent computerisation, retrieval and analysis of data, allowing comparison across units, hospitals and countries.

Current IM&T systems used in hospitals in the UK are focused on *management* information, with the use of coding and classification systems such as ICD10[2] and OPCS4.[3] *Clinical* information is either unavailable, incredibly difficult to collect and collate, or is derived from existing coding systems, and can mean different things to different people. Doctors write medical notes as part of diagnosis and treatment. At the end of the patient stay, coders interpret the notes and codify them using ICD and OPCS. The coders' interpretation of the medical notes is often different to the meaning given by the doctors. This may be because there can be many codes to choose from for each term a doctor might use. An example of this problem is shown in Box 4.1.

Box 4.1: The complexity of ICD10 codes

Typical medical description as written in the patient record:	Some of the ICD10 codes/descriptions available to match the medical description:
	I21.0 Acute transmural MI of anterior wall
	I21.1 Acute transmural MI of inferior wall
	I21.2 Acute transmural MI of other sites
	I21.3 Acute transmural MI of unspecified sites
	I21.4 Acute sub-endocardial MI
Acute MI	I21.9 Acute MI unspecified
	I22.0 Subsequent MI anterior wall
	I22.1 Subsequent MI of inferior wall
	I22.8 Subsequent MI of other sites
	I22.9 Subsequent MI of unspecified site

Box 4.2: Some medical terms for myocardial infarction

MI	Heart attack
Coronary syndrome	Cardiac event
Small MI	Large MI
Infarct	Coronary thrombosis
Inferior MI	Anterior MI

Doctors can be inconsistent in the different medical terms they use (*see* Box 4.2). This adds to the complexity of the coder's task as coders may interpret all the terms differently.

When doctors are given summarised data, the instant response is 'I have never performed this operation!' or 'I'm sure I did at least double the amount that it says here!' The problem is caused partly by the fact that the coding system was devised for epidemiological purposes rather than the collection of clinical information.

The solution, according to the Audit Commission, which carried out a study of hospital medical records in 1997, rests with the doctors:

'It is vital that doctors accept their responsibility for producing clear statements of diagnoses and procedures in the discharge letter or clinical summary.'

Setting the Records Straight (p19)[4]

The report also recommends that the requirement is recognised in consult-ant job plans, and time allowed for the activity. In reality, time is always short and clinical care is always a priority over what is still seen as administration activity; the same could be said of all aspects of record keeping. In the absence of a common healthcare language in the domain of IM&T, and inadequate systems to meet the needs of clinicians, problems remain both with the generation of data, its recording and its interpretation.

Another reason for ensuring clinical language is accurately and meaningfully codified is to support the future development of artificial intelligence in decision-support systems, by having high quality data to allow data mining and pattern recognition. This would mean that, for example, a database of millions of records could be searched for relation-ships between items of clinical information. In practical terms, it could be described as real-time research.

One way of starting the process of drawing together of the professions is via the use of a common clinical language on paper, by introducing common headings in a unified patient record.

Structure of clinical information needed for EPR

In an EPR it is essential to record clinical information in a structured way rather than as free text. According to van Bemmel and Musen[5] 'if data are not structured, the EPR is decreased to, at best, an intelligent word processor'. *Information for Health*[1] recommends the introduction of a common coding language to provide the structure needed. As previously explained, existing coding structures are not flexible enough to fulfil the need. Read Codes, a recent and more flexible system used in primary care, is better suited to the task, as it contains clinical terms as well as codes. However, in order to ensure that the system maintains its flexibility, the national strategy names the system of the future as SNOMED CT. This system combines the best of Read Codes, version 3, with SNOMED RT, a coding system developed and used in America. SNOMED CT will provide clinicians with a way of using clinical language to code rather than having to conform to a system with termin-ology meaningless to them.

Converting a paper framework into EPR via procurement specification

In Chapter 1 we state that, in order for the impact of the impending EPR to be less disruptive, a change in record-keeping practices needs to happen on paper first. We also conclude that the structure and content of a unified paper record is linked strongly to the successful implementation and use of EPR. We have mentioned in previous chapters about the advantages and disadvantages of paper ICPs when collecting and analysing clinical information. The paper UPR allows more flexibility by having standardised ways of assessing, recording and planning care and treatment, which are interchangeable and unified. In order to achieve this flexibility, it is necessary for the professions to collaborate and agree a paper framework that allows the recording of clinical information in such a way that it is easily located and useful to all concerned. This section details how experience gained from modernising the *paper* recording framework can be used to create the specification for an *electronic* record.

The implementation of a common EPR brings great challenges for working together, in particular, the need to standardise aspects of care such as record-keeping practices, which have traditionally been totally separate.

As part of the procurement for EPR, a specification is needed to cover aspects of functionality listed in *Information for Health* (*see* Figure 4.1).

If the EPR is to be patient-focused, rather than profession-focused, it needs to refer to functionality in generic terms, rather than the traditional modular approach (*see* Table 4.1).

Table 4.1: Approaches to specifying EPR functionality

Traditional approach to system specification	*Generic approach to system procurement*
Identify specialities needing EPR	Identify functions that an EPR could provide
Create modules with functions in them, depending on the clinician's preferences	Apply the functionality to patient situations such as detection of a disease, diagnosis, treatment and care and discharge

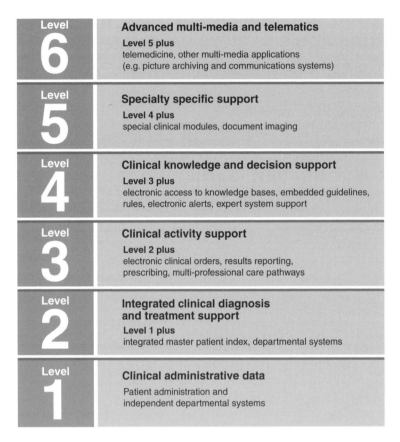

Figure 4.1 EPR levels, from *Information for Health*, Chapter 2, p37

Using the paper UPR created during the Weston project as an example, record keeping can be situated within the clinical documentation functionality of an EPR, in the following way.

1 **Assessing and recording care**: generic and specialist assessment, record of care and variation record.
2 **Planning care**: condition-specific mini-plans, care guides, medical protocols, use of problem lists.
3 **Clinical terming and coding**: unified and standardised language.
4 **Outputs**: discharge checklist, weekly discharge summary, patient information.

The Clinical Documentation section of the Pan-Bristol and Weston EPR Specification, created in 2002 as part of procurement, is structured in this way.

Decision support/evidence into practice

We cannot go into detail about the complexities of decision-support systems in a book about record keeping. However, there is a potential link between the evidence-base within the UPR, and the future functionality of an EPR.

Electronic decision-support systems can be defined as:

'active knowledge systems which use two or more items of data to generate patient-specific advice.'

Handbook of Medical Informatics (p262)[5]

With the growing body of knowledge generated by advances in healthcare, it is unrealistic to expect a healthcare professional to remember everything required to make clinical decisions. Using decision support within an EPR *actively* supports decision making, rather than the clinician needing recall, or to seek knowledge *before* being able to weigh up the options. In order to inform the future development of decision-support systems, work needs to be done on what knowledge a system should contain. The work carried out within the Weston UPR to create care guides has the potential to inform the content of an electronic multiprofessional decision-support system.

Finally . . .

This chapter has provided an insight into the links between paper and electronic records and the extra benefits computerised systems can bring. However, the culture change needed to take on the challenge of EPR is enormous, not least in the way healthcare professionals use information. An appreciation of the basics of information handling is also needed if we are to maximise the potential of the EPR, and make full use of *all* the functionality on offer. The next chapter focuses on modern healthcare information needs in terms of key issues in the management and use of information, which are based around record keeping.

References

1   Burns F (1998) *Information for Health: an information strategy for the modern NHS 1998–2005*. Department of Health Publications, Wetherby.
2   World Health Organization (1992) *International Classification of Diseases, version 10*. WHO, Geneva.

3   South-west Regional Health Authority (1992) *Operations and Procedures Classification, version 4*. HMSO, London.
4   Audit Commission (1997) *Setting the Records Straight*. HMSO, London.
5   van Bemmel JH and Musen MA (1997) *Handbook of Medical Informatics*. Springer-Verlag, Heidelberg.

5

Uses of the information within a patient record

The Audit Commission reports that clinical professionals spend about 25% of their time collecting data on their patients.[1] We mentioned in Chapter 1 that traditional paper records often have information within them that is repetitive, complex and incomplete. It therefore seems that clinicians may be wasting their time recording information that is not fulfilling the needs of a modern health service, or the patients it serves.

This chapter starts by delving into the recent history of the collection, use and management of information in the NHS. The NHS is subject to constant change; this has major implications for the way in which information is gathered and used to support healthcare. Implementation of *The NHS Plan*[2] requires a fundamental change in culture – that is, thinking, practice and delivery of healthcare over the next ten years.[3] The deliverables outlined in *Information for Health*[4] are a vital and underpinning part of the modernisation agenda. The change in thinking required to be able to adopt new information practices such as EPR, and let go of established beliefs and values, constitutes a huge challenge for NHS professionals.

The use of aggregated information in healthcare was first accentuated with the introduction of clinical audit. It was an attempt to ensure that clinical care was measured, and to provide a basis for assessing improvements.[5] Unfortunately, all but the most forward thinking of clinicians saw audit as a bolt-on activity, not related to the core activity of looking after patients.[6] Audit meetings were secret events, with the need to keep all data confidential, and there was no sharing of findings or lessons learnt. This meant that information that would have been vital in pinpointing problems in care, for example with the Bristol babies, went either uncollected or unrecognised by the managers who could have attempted to resolve situations as they arose. The recent publication of the official investigation of the Bristol babies case confirms this.[7]

The publication of the *first* national health information strategy in the early 1990s[8] had the potential to ensure that information was moved to the top of the NHS agenda, but it failed to engage the interest of most clinicians. With the advent of clinical governance in 1997, the importance of good information was again highlighted, with a call to implement:

'a comprehensive programme of quality improvement activities which includes effective monitoring of clinical care with high quality systems for clinical record keeping and the collection of relevant information.'
A First Class Service (p379)[9]

For the first time, trust chief executives were made responsible for *acting on* information. However, the collection, collation and interpretation of clinical information continued to rest with the clinicians, with:

'full participation by all hospital doctors in audit programmes, including national external audit programmes endorsed by the Commission for Health Improvement.'
A First Class Service (p36)[9]

The impact of the highly publicised clinical mistakes of the late 1990s has been to reduce the status of clinicians, and doctors in particular, in the eyes of the public. In order to restore public confidence, there is a need to share and be open with information about clinical performance. Clinical governance has reinforced the ideal of working in partnership with the patient.[9] The need to manage risk by giving the patient informed choice about treatment has engendered amongst some clinicians a strong desire for access to up-to-date, accurate performance statistics available during consultation.

The creation of the Centre for Health Improvement (CHI), with its right to access evidence about clinical practice and visit trusts to ask probing questions about standards, has helped to ensure that clinicians pay attention to their own practice, and that of their team. Evidence about standards is difficult to access. Clinical record keeping *should* contain relevant audit information. Until now, audit information has often been collected separately in an attempt to provide uniform data about some areas of practice; current record keeping does not support *either* a standardised approach amenable to audit, *or* an integrated view of clinical practice.

Intensive and time-consuming preparation is needed to provide details of care treatment activity and outcomes for CHI visits. This has become another driver for the adoption of ICPs. However, with the growing realisation of the difficulty paper ICPs cause, the increased flexibility provided by a paper UPR seems an ideal interim solution. The UPR has an added benefit, as discussed in previous chapters, of informing the specification for EPR, and preparing staff for change.

This chapter continues by looking at the uses of the data that is collected in traditional records, and how a paper UPR could be the forerunner of an electronic record that fulfils future information needs.

Box 5.1: The uses of information in clinical records

- A record of care and treatment.
- A communication medium.
- To show professionalism.
- A quality assurance tool.
- Defence against complaints.
- 'An elaborate accounting mechanism.'[10]

Traditional paper records have many uses in today's health service (*see* Box 5.1). Information is the most important resource a hospital holds, according to the Audit Commission.[1] However, if traditional paper records are not providing the best way of harnessing the information collected and stored within, then the move to EPR must be preceded by an in-depth examination of the structure and function of the record, the framework it uses to collect and store information, and the methods in use to extract aggregated information. This will ensure that the *Information for Health* principle of obtaining management information as a by-product of clinical information is taken on board.

The design of the Weston UPR has attempted to make the best use of the information within a patient record by ensuring that it is collected and stored in a standardised way at the point of care, so that it can be easily extracted at a later date.

Clinical governance

A key part of clinical governance is the use of *clinical* information – collecting it, storing it, analysing and using it. In our experience, *data* often means computers and numbers to those directly concerned with clinical care. *Information*, on the other hand, is data that has been interpreted and can be used to some benefit when thinking about quality of care. However, information is useless unless the data it comes from is of good quality. The Kennedy Report[7] – the result of the public inquiry into the events with the Bristol heart babies – found that Bristol was 'awash with data'. Recommendation number 148 of the report says that a 'single approach to collecting data should be adopted, which clinicians can trust and use, and from which information about both clinical and administrative performance can be derived'. This statement matches the principle of deriving management information from clinical information.

The Audit Commission[11] makes the point that:

*'improvement requires the active involvement not only of the chief executive but also of non-executive directors and other directors, **and** of clinicians and managers who – whether or not they have become involved with data quality issues – ultimately generate and should be making use of the information that exists.'*

Data Remember[11]

So it seems to us that the key to clinical governance, and to being comfortable with clinical accountability, is the changing of professional culture to embrace informatics – the generation, storage and use of information.

Clinical governance assumes the use of evidence-based clinical guidelines. One example of this is the NICE guideline for Pressure Ulcer Risk Assessment and Prevention.[12] Implementation of such a guideline seems like a good idea, but how do you know it's being used, and that it improves care? One way to find out if it is working is to measure adherence, as recommended in the document. Point 5.6 says:

'prospective clinical audit programmes should record the extent to which care adheres to the guideline. Such programmes are more likely to be effective in improving patient care when they form part of the organisation's formal clinical governance arrangements.'

Pressure Ulcer Risk Assessment and Prevention[12]

But why not go further, and evaluate the *outcome* of the measures put in place as a result of the guideline? Measurement of outcomes is always difficult, but a simple way of measuring pressure sore incidence would be a good place to start. From our experience on the wards and working in clinical audit, we know that this type of data collection can be time-consuming, and fraught with duplication and inaccuracy.

An example of improved information practice

Using the GPP, pressure sore information is collected at the bedside as part of clinical assessment. This information is used by anyone looking after the patient, including the patient and carers. When the patient is discharged the data within the patient record is filed in the notes for the coders to see.

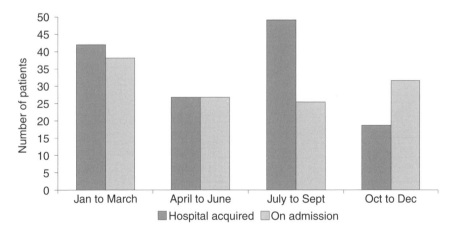

Figure 5.1 Pressure sore incidence 2001

Figure 5.1 shows information taken directly from the coded data at Weston. This is just a simple summary of the information collected directly at the point of care, as part of care, but in reality, the data can be presented to show where incidence has decreased or increased in response to implementation of a guideline, for example. It can show up hotspots where extra resources are needed. Within the NHS, this type of information is commonly collected already – the difference is that the UPR allows this to be collected as part of the care process, not as an extra to normal record keeping. This is just a small example of the potential of information collected at the point of care, stored and used effectively to become the basis of some elements of clinical governance.

The pressure sore information example illustrates one aspect of making better use of clinical record keeping to audit practice. This could apply to any aspect of practice that is included within a UPR – collection of information for National Service Frameworks, monitoring health and safety issues involved with moving and handling patients, ensuring that patients' nutritional needs are met, or any aspect of care where best practice guidance is used. The NMC guidelines for Records and Record-keeping[13] state that the quality of record keeping is also a reflection of the quality of professional practice. This practical information-based approach to record keeping is one way of ensuring that audit is not a bolt-on activity, but an integral part of the way clinicians work.

Answering complaints

Before the UPR came into being, answering a complaint from the clinical documentation was a time-consuming and laborious process. Information was often incomplete, and duplication meant that parts of the record gave the same type of information in a different way. Routine aspects of care often cause complaints. Aspects such as patients' hygiene and nutrition were often unrecorded, so the complaint could not be answered.

The following case study is based on a real complaint answered with the use of the information collected within the recording framework of the UPR. It was easy to cross-reference the GPP and daily record of care with the information on the variation record. For example, on page 55, response to the assertion about Mr Smith's eating was answered fully. Answering a complaint in the way shown in Table 5.1 also allows improvements to the recording framework and the evidence base behind it.

Mr Smith was an elderly gentleman who was admitted for routine surgery. Following discharge, the family became concerned about his general health.

His condition continued to deteriorate and resulted in his re-admission to hospital. Mr Smith died during this admission. The family wrote a letter of complaint, which included the following points about hospital care.

1 Nobody seemed to care if he was eating or not.
2 Food intake not recorded.
3 Father's dentures were not cleaned.

Table 5.1 The response compiled from the patient record

No.	Question	Response	Source of response	Comments about the record
1	Nobody seemed to care if he was eating or not.	Mr Smith was assessed daily by nursing staff regarding his ability to eat and his appetite. The records show that he had an acceptable intake when his appetite was good. On the days his appetite was poor, the fluid charts show that on occasions he refused diet and fluids.	GPP for assessment of appetite. Daily record asks the question. Fluid charts.	Possible change to GPP required to expand assessment. Food chart would have been better practice. Nutritional assessment would have been helpful.
2	Food intake not recorded.	The daily record of care shows that meals were eaten. The fluid charts describe which foods were eaten and when foods were refused.	Daily record. Fluid charts.	Use of waitresses for nutrition would allow complete recording if they are trained to use the record. Nutrition care guide could have been implemented.
3	Father's dentures were not cleaned.	The records show that Mr Smith received regular mouthcare. Staff follow the trust care guide for mouthcare, which clearly states the procedure to assist patients when cleaning dentures.	Daily record. Care guides.	Need to make sure that care guides are ratified and policy updated to reflect care guides. All nurses must sign to say they have read the care guides.

Thompson and Wright[14]

Using UPR information to improve referrals

In our experience, the process of referral between clinical areas relies on the judgement of individual clinicians. This often results in a subjective view of the patient's suitability for referral, which causes confusion and delays. A mechanism for supporting referral was discovered in the GPP during the pilot phase of the Weston project. The modified Barthel score on page 2 of the document provides an objective assessment of stroke patients' fitness for transfer from acute care to rehabilitation unit. A score of 10 or above seemed to be key, so this was accepted by both clinical areas as a satisfactory method of assessing readiness for transfer. The assessment has also added clarity to the readiness of acute patients to transfer to Weston's interim care setting. It allows a history of improvements in function to be used to judge suitability for transfer. The same information, which is collected daily as part of assessment, has been used by medical teams to measure outcomes at three points during the patient stay. This is a powerful example of how one piece of information, routinely collected, can be used in a variety of ways.

Finally . . .

Information for Health represents the ideal view of the NHS of the future. The reality is that its history, the autonomy of many of its staff and the politics involved with its modernisation combine to form a huge barrier to that idealism. However, in order for the EPR to work best, attention needs to be paid to clinicians' understanding and use of all types of work-related information from the clinicians' point of view. Record keeping continues to be vitally important, but is often seen as a boring and tedious part of practice. In the future, computerised records will be a reality, and real-time, high quality data a necessity. For both clinical and non-clinical staff to record high quality data, they need to appreciate the importance of the information they collect and of its use in aggregated form, as well as in individual patient care. In the next chapter, the importance of effective change management is explained, with examples of strategies used and lessons learnt during the implementation of the Weston project.

References

1   Audit Commission (1995) *For Your Information – a study of information management and systems in the acute hospital*. HMSO, London.

2   NHS Executive (2000) *The NHS Plan*. Department of Health, London.
3   Iles V and Sutherland K (2001) *Organisational Change – a review for healthcare managers, professionals and researchers*. National Co-ordinating Centre for NHS Service Delivery and Organisation R&D, London.
4   Burns F (1998) *Information for Health: an information strategy for the modern NHS 1998–2005*. Department of Health Publications, Wetherby.
5   Department of Health (1989) *Working for Patients*. HMSO, London.
6   Johnson G, Davies HAO and Crombie IK (2000) Improving care or professional advantage? What makes clinicians do audit and how do they fare? *Health Bulletin*. **58**(4): 276–85.
7   Bristol Royal Infirmary Inquiry (2001) *Learning from Bristol: the report of the public inquiry into children's heart surgery at Bristol Royal Infirmary 1984–1995*. HMSO, London.
8   NHS Management Executive (1992) *Getting Better with Information*. Available at www.doh.gov.uk/ipu/strategy/archive/1992/index.htm.
9   Department of Health (1997) *A First Class Service: quality in the new NHS*. HMSO, London.
10   Allen D (1998) Record keeping and routine nursing practice: a view from the wards. *J Adv Nurs*. **27**: 1223–30.
11   Audit Commission (2002) *Data Remember – improving the quality of patient-based information in the NHS*. Audit Commission, London.
12   National Institute for Clinical Excellence (2001) *Inherited Guideline for Pressure Ulcer Risk Assessment and Prevention*. NICE, London.
13   Nursing and Midwifery Council (2002) *Guidelines for Records and Record-keeping*. NMC, London.
14   Thompson D and Wright K (2001) *Complaints Case Study*. Weston Area Health Trust. Unpublished.

6

Managing change

'The NHS Plan *sets out a completely new way of delivering healthcare. At a local level success is totally dependent on change management. There must be an active managerial role in resolving the problems and providing the resources to successfully apply information and IT in healthcare. In this climate the NHS must take every opportunity to share best practice and demonstrate real innovation.*

We need to create an environment of innovation by encouraging new ideas, sharing good practice and managing the risks. The purpose of innovating through information and IT is to transform the business processes. For the NHS this translates to new clinical practices and information flows and processes. The step change required by The NHS Plan, *the expectations of patients and the public, and the pace of technological change demand a new approach to innovation. Standardisation and mandating will be required for key services and in key areas but innovation must be encouraged too. The best ideas can then be shared, adopted and taken forward for the whole NHS.'*

Building the Information Core[1]

In this chapter, we describe some of the characteristics of change. This includes a review of clinical projects resulting in successful change. We also give examples of strategies and models that can be used in the implementation and subsequent evolution of UPR.

Characteristics of change

Change is a difficult concept to describe. Iles and Sutherland[2] explain the characteristics of change as:

- **planned**: a product of conscious reasoning and actions, where people know why change is needed, what needs to happen, and what the result will be
- **emergent**: apparently spontaneous and unplanned. Sometimes things appear to happen out of the blue, unrelated to another change, or as a result of external factors.

In order to manage change effectively, it seems necessary to identify, explore and challenge people's assumptions. We need to understand that organisational change is a process that can be facilitated by perceptive and insightful planning and analysis. Well-crafted, sensitive implementation phases are needed, while acknowledging that change can never be fully isolated from the effects of serendipity, uncertainty and chance.

Change can occur in the following ways.

- Episodic change can often involve the replacement of one strategy with another. An example of this might be the decision to change from testing gastric aspirate with litmus paper to testing with pH sensitive strips, in response to appraisal of evidence. It takes place in one go, and is done.
- Continuous change is characterised by people constantly adapting and editing ideas they get from different sources. Together, these smaller initiatives happening at the same time can create substantial change. An example of this might be the ongoing updating and implementing of individual care guides by small groups of clinicians. The effect would be continual improving and updating of practice.

The types of change listed below are identified in change management literature and have the characteristics we have just described.

- Developmental change can be planned or emergent and often focuses on the improvement of a skill or process – learning to surf the Internet, for example.
- Transitional change is planned and episodic. Lewin's transitional change theory involves unfreezing, moving and refreezing behaviour.[3] Prince project management seems to fit this method of change.[4]
- Transformational change is also episodic in nature. It requires a shift in assumptions made by the organisation and its members, and can result in an organisation that continually learns, adapts and improves. For example, response to risk management issues may need this sort of approach to ensure organisation-wide behavioural change.

This way of categorising change makes it seem a rational, controlled and orderly process but, in our experience, organisational change is usually extremely complex and filled with unexpected twists and turns. Even the most carefully planned change can be both challenging and perplexing for all involved.

Culture change within the clinical professions

In order to understand how a change in thinking can be achieved and sustained in the complex setting of the NHS, it is useful to explore:

- the ways in which professionals recognise the need for change and achieve change within the working environment
- existing initiatives which have been successful in achieving change in healthcare settings
- how the above methods can be used to achieve change within the *Information for Health* agenda.

The need to ensure that clinicians change to meet the needs of the techno-logical changes within *Information for Health* is clearly stated at the begin-ning of this chapter. The idea that clinicians will take on board the need for change from an IM&T perspective is unrealistic and doomed to failure. In the clinical world of many and conflicting priorities, clinicians' perceptions of patient-centred issues take priority. The question to be asked is what makes clinicians want to change clinical practice, and how do they achieve it in complex clinical settings?

A review of the professional literature about changing practice gives an idea of incentives for change and tools used by clinicians to achieve changes in practice.

The literature reviewed was from 1997 to 2001 and covers the profes-sions listed in Box 6.1.

Box 6.1: Professions discussed in the literature

- Nursing – paediatrics, critical care, mental health, orthopaedics, specialist nurses.
- Midwifery and obstetrics.
- Multiprofessional teams.
- Community services.
- Nursing education.
- Clinical managers.

The review looked at changes to practice, rather than change management itself, in order to isolate what caused the change. The variety of methods and ideas were used to show that change was needed, including:

- investigation of risk management issues[5]
- need to implement National Service Frameworks[6]
- participatory action research with bedside nurses[7]
- the influence of carrying out clinical audit and comparing data[8]
- desire to implement evidence-based practice[9]
- mutual recognition of the need to change.[10]

Box 6.2: Factors that made practice change

- Transformational leadership skills.[11]
- The benefit of multidisciplinary linkages.[5]
- The use of 'implementer consensus'.[12]
- Action research.[7,13]
- The idea for the change came from the clinical team.[11,12]
- Lengthy and detailed planning increased confidence.[14]
- Clear communications channels.[11]
- Measured benefits of using a care pathway made obvious.[13]

Even if the conditions are right for change, this does not mean that the process is easy. Several barriers are highlighted in the literature (*see* Box 6.3).

Box 6.3: Barriers to change

- Professional apathy.[15]
- Organisational difficulties clinicians are faced with when carrying out changes.[8]
- Constraining influences exerted by clinical managers, from budgetary allocations to failure to use position and authority to influence change.[8]

It seems from this review that early involvement of clinicians increases the likelihood of change lasting. Plant provides evidence to support this assumption.[16] In the Weston project, it was agreed by key clinicians early on that a unified record should be designed to improve communication, reduce workload and improve standards of patient care through evidence-based practice. This may have contributed to the success of the change.

The context of change

It is evident that there can be many factors to consider, so change must be seen in context. This section gives an overview of models that can be used to help manage the type of changes described in this book. There are many other approaches to both organisational and culture change management. Iles and Sutherland have published an excellent review of tools, models and approaches, including evidence of their success in changing practice.[2] This is intended to 'bridge the gap between the commitment to change and action' and illustrates the possibilities for achievement of change.

'Systems thinking' reflects organisations like the NHS which have complex networks of inter-relationships. A system is made up of related and interdependent parts, so that any system may be viewed as a whole. It cannot be considered in isolation from its environment. A system which is in equilibrium will change only if some type of energy is applied. Players within a system have a view of that system's function and purpose, and players' views may be very different from each other.[2]

One way of ensuring a whole systems approach to change is by applying **PESTLE**, a model to help break down the organisational environment to reveal factors within the whole system.[17]

A **PESTLE** analysis of the UPR is shown in Box 6.4.

Box 6.4: PESTLE analysis of the UPR

Political	Government policy, white papers, political short-termism.
Economic	Budgetary constraints, population changes.
Social	Greater involvement of patients/clients in clinical decisions.
Technological	New IT systems, medical devices, lab tests.
Legal	Specific legislation – nurse prescribing, specific litigation causes media interest, risk management.
Ethical	Patient choice, eligibility requirements for access to new services, quality of patient information, professional standards.

Prior to planning change a SWOT analysis can be completed. SWOT is an acronym for Strengths, Weaknesses, Opportunities and Threats and can be used to identify those associated with the proposed change. The idea of this model is to maximise strengths and opportunities, whilst minimising threats and weaknesses, wherever possible. For an example of how this might work when analysing the UPR, *see* Box 6.5.

Box 6.5: SWOT analysis related to UPR

Strengths	Weaknesses
Multidisciplinary working. Standardised approach. Improved communication Evidence-based practice. Expert resource for patients and colleagues. Improved risk management. Patient focus.	Lack of resources. Availability of all disciplines. Strength of professional boundaries. Lack of ownership of the concept.
Opportunities	**Threats**
Improved patient outcomes. Increasing knowledge. Developing protocols. New ways of working to move towards EPR.	Lack of resources. Coordinating the change. Learning experience. Risk to patient care, whilst making changes to practice.

This analysis reveals that the strengths and opportunities outweigh the threats and weaknesses.

To reinforce the findings of the SWOT analysis, a force field analysis can also be undertaken. Empirical research suggests that following a force field analysis it is more effective to adopt strategies that will reduce the resistant forces rather than efforts to increase the driving ones.[18] The originator of this well-respected model was Lewin in 1951.[3] Figure 6.1 shows a force field analysis of UPR development.

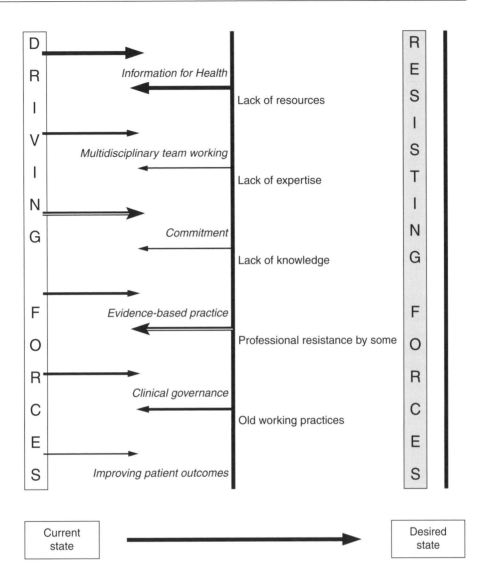

Figure 6.1 Force field analysis of UPR development

SWOT and the force field analysis were applied retrospectively to the Weston project to illustrate to the reader the benefits of having an overall view before implementing change. However, the factors listed in Box 6.5 and Figure 6.1 were revealed to us when we reviewed the project to show other organisations how we achieved the change. These were the lessons we learnt during the project.

1 **Vision**. It has been helpful to have a vision of how things need to be in the future. The promise of the EPR, and the need for cultural change to be able to use it, has ensured that some of the practical steps needed to move towards the vision have been put in place.

2 **Planning**. A huge amount of planning took place over the four years of the project. Although project-planning methodology, such as Prince,[4] was not used *per se*, elements such as stages and timescales were vital in ensuring that change occurred. The use of tools such as Lewin and SWOT would have enhanced our view of the project.

3 **Evaluation**. The use of audit results and information gained from trust systems was key in raising awareness of current practice, as well as feeding back results of hard work to the teams who initiated the change. Some results gave the project a real boost, added to its commitment to the next stage, and helped sustain changes that were made.

4 **Communication**. This was the hardest part of the project to maintain. Multidisciplinary group meetings were essential to allow people to understand each other's point of view. The process of building an ICP facilitated communication by process mapping the patient journey in detail, thus getting every member of the group to contribute. Huge and continuing effort was required to ensure that everyone knew current status of the changes and some idea of what was to come.

5 **Ownership**. The importance of ownership is shown in the commitment of the pilot ward to making the UPR work, contrasted with the disinterest in updating handover practice on two of the rollout wards. The Documentation Link Group has strong ownership of the UPR and this has been invaluable in progressing and evaluating change. However, ownership can also be a threat. Experience during this project has shown that those who have ownership of a past change sometimes obstruct future changes. The key may be in developing staff to alter the culture of the organisation to one that continuously learns, adapts and improves.

6 **Other drivers**. Several initiatives helped to push the pace of change, including clinical governance,[14] *Information for Health*,[19] Audit Commission and Royal Colleges audit programmes and Clinical Negligence Scheme for Trusts (CNST) accreditation.[20]

7 The combination of top-down and bottom-up approaches has ensured involvement of staff, along with the highlighting of issues such as individual professional accountability. Board-level direction was provided by ratification of Trustwide Policies and Guidelines, whilst opinions of frontline staff were actively sought and incorporated into

the UPR as it evolved. At times, this included compromising on the little things to ensure continued ownership.

In previous chapters, we stressed the importance of the patient-focused approach to developing a UPR. This is also an effective strategy for change. It provides a means of bringing diverse disciplines together as a team to review evidence and put it into practice, taking the focus away from each single profession.[21] This approach lessens arguments about whose opinion is most valued.

The models mentioned in this section are well tested and can prove effective in examining current systems with a complex organisation. The next section looks at strategies that can be adopted to support them.

Strategies to support change

In this section we give examples of strategies we have found helpful in initiating, implementing and maintaining change.

Raising awareness

An example of where raising awareness has lowered resistance to change and encouraged people to get involved is the use of demonstrations in the EPR procurement process. Clinical *and* non-clinical staff who have been involved in Pan-Bristol and Weston system evaluation are beginning to see the relevance of the changes made to record keeping at Weston, in the context of the EPR.

Another factor, which helped bring about awareness of the need for change, was the use of the *Information for Health* video,[22] distributed via an Information Resource Pack produced by Avon Professional Advisory Group (APAG). The connection of the vision with reality may have helped to lower some of the resistance to change.

Awareness was also raised by the use of:

• record-keeping roadshows
• poster and splat campaigns

- explanation of benefits, including less duplication and less writing
- work-based training
- project manager involvement at a practice level.

The following points are more practical, but were useful in tackling resistance to the changes taking place.

1 No system can solve the problem of poor quality recording of care.
2 Electronic systems rely on the use of guidelines and rules.
3 There is no point in changing the documentation unless we can move it forward.
4 Recording every aspect of the patient's care every time it happens is unrealistic (audit has shown this many times).
5 To focus too much on recording every aspect of complex care will ensure that the new patient record is merely the nursing process by another name.
6 To record *variations* from the care detailed in care guides is the only way of sifting what is special about the patient – good risk management practice.

Process mapping

Process mapping is an established tool for change management but is fairly new to the NHS. It is becoming widely used via the Booked Admissions programme and Modernisation Agency. More detail about how it works can be found at www.doh.gsi.gov.uk/modernisation. We have found process mapping extremely useful in raising awareness of the need for change and revealing the number of people involved.

Sustaining change

Ongoing training in the use and completion of a UPR is vital to the successful *embedding* of change. Even if huge efforts are made during the rollout of changes, and all staff have access to initial training, ongoing training is often more problematic, due to limited resources and conflicting priorities.

Feedback of audit results is vital in letting people know that the change

is working. It also allows people to feed in ideas for ongoing improvement of the UPR.

There is a need for clinical champions to learn together about change in
order to build up a local knowledge base for use within trusts and give
mutual support. At Weston, a variety of forums exist, giving clinicians the
opportunity to work together and keep up communication.

National initiatives to promote change

The NHSIA has set up a series of Informatics Learning Networks (ILN)
across the country.[23] The ILNs are designed to help people learn about
informatics in order to promote cultural change in the NHS. Methods of
learning are a combination of:

- organised learning forums, with speakers and workshops
- an interactive website, where participants can look at other activities
  across the country and access resources to help them
- Local Learning Groups, consisting of 10–12 colleagues who get
  together to work on a work-based informatics problem such as, for
  example, how to deliver clinical governance information.

The ILNs are an ideal way of facilitating learning about change within
the clinical arena, but related to IM&T. It makes resources accessible to
larger numbers of clinical change agents and provides peer support to
help overcome organisational difficulties and professional apathy –
cited in the literature as the main reasons for failure to achieve and
maintain change. The use of a virtual learning network, via the
website, allows people to participate without travelling if they have
access to NHSnet.

Coping with restraints

The NHS will always be short of staff and short of money. As part of
the review of the Weston project, neighbouring trusts requested information about staffing levels at the time of the change. They were
worried that their limited resources would lead to failure of the same
project in their areas. However, sickness levels at Weston were
unusually high during the first three months of the change. Also, the

project took place with no additional funding, other than the presence of a practice development nurse who acted as project manager. The leadership and commitment of this one person was the driving force that overcame the restraints and ensured the continued engagement of clinical staff. The whole team should therefore be credited, against the odds, with the success of the UPR. However, better resources could have accelerated the process.

Recommendations

It is essential to bear in mind some high level principles, to ensure that ownership does not get in the way of objectivity. The following principles have helped to smooth progress in the Weston project and ensure object-ivity of decision making about changes.

1   Management information should be derived from clinical informa-tion.
2   Information flows should be mapped according to the patient journey.
3   Attention should be paid to the 'interfaces' between wards/depart-ments.
4   Changes to the way care is recorded are inevitable.
5   Changes to the way care is delivered are welcome, as long as they benefit the patient and the information flow.

There is a need to bridge the gap between the IM&T and clinical worlds, as well as ensuring growing communication between the professions. A change management plan for the modernising of clinical informatics through changes in record keeping, linking to the change plan for EPR, should incorporate lessons learnt both from professional experience and current change initiatives.

As part of implementing *any* change, we would recommend that existing knowledge, such as the review mentioned above, and the materials/training should be utilised more fully. Local clinical change agents should be identified, and given the incentive to push forward the informatics change agenda from the clinical perspective. This could be achieved using drivers such as continuing professional development, risk management and clinical governance.

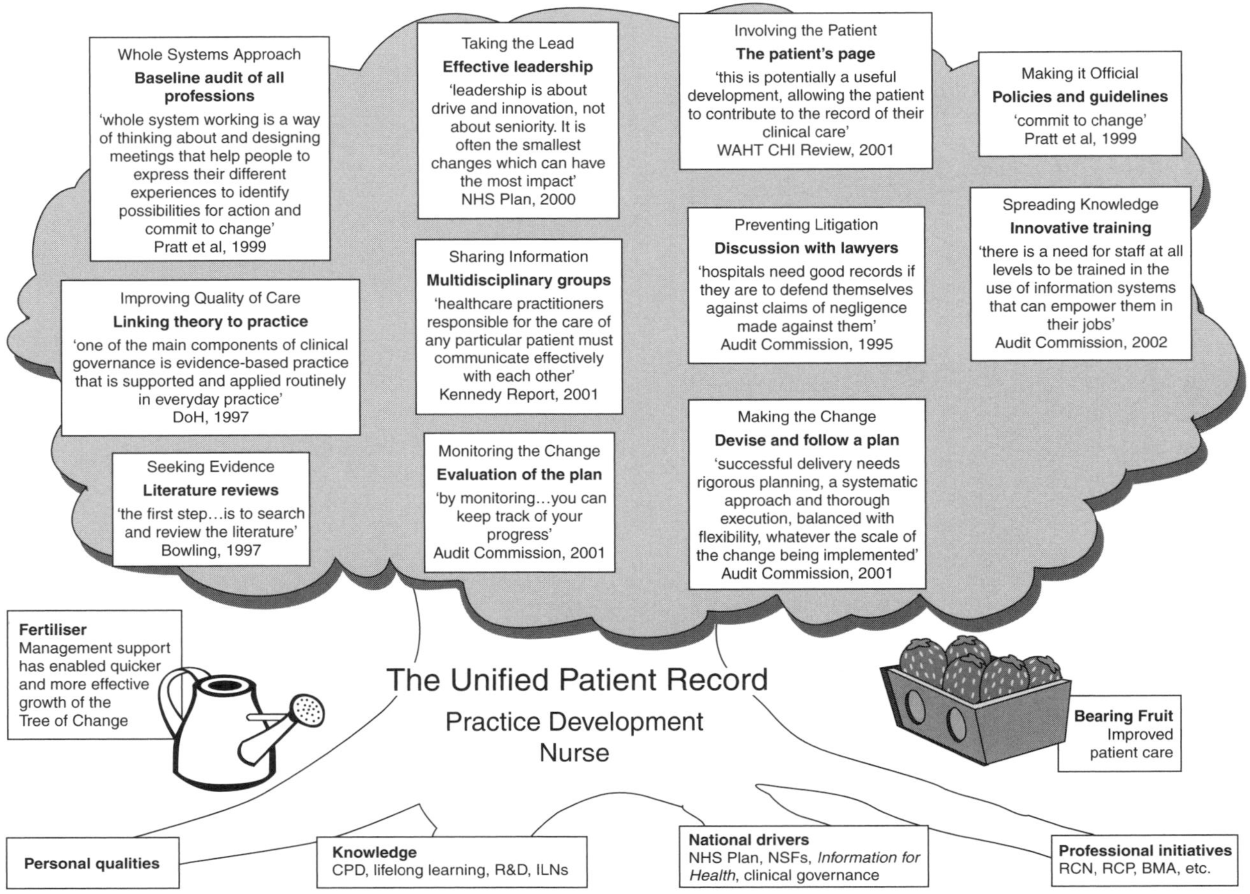

Figure 6.2 The Tree of Change applied to the UPR[24]

Making it Official
Policies and guidelines
'commit to change'
Pratt et al, 1999

Spreading Knowledge
Innovative training
'there is a need for staff at all
levels to be trained in the
use of information systems
that can empower them in
their jobs'
Audit Commission, 2002

Involving the Patient
The patient's page
'this is potentially a useful
development, allowing the patient
to contribute to the record of their
clinical care'
WAHT CHI Review, 2001

Preventing Litigation
Discussion with lawyers
'hospitals need good records if
they are to defend themselves
against claims of negligence
made against them'
Audit Commission, 1995

Making the Change
Devise and follow a plan
'successful delivery needs
rigorous planning, a systematic
approach and thorough
execution, balanced with
flexibility, whatever the scale of
the change being implemented'
Audit Commission, 2001

Taking the Lead
Effective leadership
'leadership is about
drive and innovation, not
about seniority. It is
often the smallest
changes which can have
the most impact'
NHS Plan, 2000

Sharing Information
Multidisciplinary groups
'healthcare practitioners
responsible for the care of
any particular patient must
communicate effectively
with each other'
Kennedy Report, 2001

Monitoring the Change
Evaluation of the plan
'by monitoring…you can
keep track of your
progress'
Audit Commission, 2001

Whole Systems Approach
**Baseline audit of all
professions**
'whole system working is a way
of thinking about and designing
meetings that help people to
express their different
experiences to identify
possibilities for action and
commit to change'
Pratt et al, 1999

Improving Quality of Care
Linking theory to practice
'one of the main components of clinical
governance is evidence-based practice
that is supported and applied routinely
in everyday practice'
DoH, 1997

Seeking Evidence
Literature reviews
'the first step…is to search
and review the literature'
Bowling, 1997

The Unified Patient Record
Practice Development
Nurse

Bearing Fruit
Improved
patient care

Professional initiatives
RCN, RCP, BMA, etc.

National drivers
NHS Plan, NSFs, *Information for
Health*, clinical governance

Knowledge
CPD, lifelong learning, R&D, ILNs

Personal qualities

Fertiliser
Management support
has enabled quicker
and more effective
growth of the
Tree of Change

Finally . . .

Unless existing healthcare professionals understand the importance of the information they routinely collect, they will not recognise the deficiencies in present systems. This means that they will not see, for example:

- the benefits of changing practices to enable clinical information to be collected as part of everyday record keeping via an electronic patient record
- the usefulness of their information to them when easily accessed in aggregated form for clinical governance, research and patient case load management.

To describe the many facets involved in this type of project, we produced a model for practice development, called the Tree of Change.[24] This model was originally created to illustrate service development in tissue viability and was presented at an international conference. We chose a tree to represent the way in which an idea can take root and grow and, since its conception, it has become apparent that the model can be effective, applied to any type of practice development. The model displays that nurses are in the ideal position to effect change – commitment, enthusiasm and knowledge are necessary elements to enable development of the individual; nurturing by responsive managers leads to the growth of the Tree of Change. Figure 6.2 shows its application to UPR.

References

1   NHS Executive (2001) *Building the Information Core: implementing the NHS Plan*. NHS Executive, Leeds.
2   Iles V and Sutherland K (2001) *Managing Change in the NHS*. National Co-ordinating Centre for NHS Service Delivery and Organisation R&D, London.
3   Lewin K (1951) *Field Theory in Social Science*. Harper and Row, New York.
4   Prince2 Project Management. www.prince2.com
5   Morison B and Baker C (2001) Tissue viability: how to raise the awareness of pressure sore prevention. *Br J Midwif.* **9**(3): 147–50.
6   Cotter A (2001) Improving services for older people. *Prof Nurse.* **16**(5): 11–32.
7   Suderman EM, Deatrich JV, Johnson LS and Sawatsky-Dickson DM (2000) Action research sets the stage to improve discharge preparation. *Paediatr Nurs.* **26**(6): 571–6, 583–4.
8   Johnson D, Davies HAO and Crombie IK (2000) Improving care or profes-

sional advantage? What makes clinicians do audit and how do they fare? *Health Bulletin.* **58**(4): 276–85.

9 Kneale J (2000) Evidence-based practice in orthopaedic nursing. *J Orthopaed Nurs.* **4**(1): 16–21

10 Williamson SH and Hutcherson C (1998) Mutual recognition: response to the regulatory implications of a changing healthcare environment. *Adv Prac Nurs Quart.* **4**(3): 86–93.

11 Manley K (2000) Organisational culture and consultant nurse outcomes. *Nurs Crit Care.* **5**(4): 179–86.

12 Burrell G and Rush J (1998) Implementaing self-medication in an ortho-paedic rehabilitation unit. *J Orthopaed Nurs.* **2**(3): 136–40.

13 Underwood F and Parker J (1998) Developing and evaluating an acute stroke care pathway through action research. *Nurse Res.* **6**(2): 27–38.

14 Department of Health (1997) *The New NHS: modern, dependable.* HMSO, London.

15 Page S and Meerabeau L (2000) Achieving change through reflective practice: closing the loop. *Nurs Edu Today.* **20**(5): 365–72.

16 Plant R (1987) *Managing Change and Making it Stick.* Gower Publishing, Aldershot.

17 National Health Service Training Division (1994) *Meeting the Challenge of Change.* NHSTD, Bristol.

18 Zand D (1995) Force field analysis. In: N Nicholson (ed.) *Encyclopaedic Dictionary of Organisational Behaviour.* Blackwell, Oxford.

19 Burns F (1998) *Information for Health: an information strategy for the modern NHS 1998–2005.* Department of Health Publications, Wetherby.

20 Clinical Negligence Scheme for Trusts (1999) Risk Management Standards.

21 Currell R, Wainright P and Urquart C (2000) *Nursing Record Systems: effects on nursing practice and healthcare outcomes* (*Cochrane Review*). The Cochrane Library, Issue 4. Update Software, Oxford.

22 *Information for Health* (1998) Video by NHSIA.

23 NHSIA Informatics Learning Network. www.nhsia.nhs.uk/nhid

24 Thompson D and Wright K (1995) *The Tree of Change.* 5th European Conference on Advances in Wound Management. Conference Proceedings. Macmillan, London.

7

Frequently asked questions

If we write less, are we still 'covering our backs'? Because standardised recording frameworks are provided, it is easier to confirm the care given rather than needing to think about devising individualised plans from scratch. It takes less time to write, so there's more chance of records being complete. Writing concisely and with implicit guidelines is much better than not writing at all. In a court of law, if it is not documented, it hasn't been done.

Where do we write? The essentials of care are predicted and built in to the record, so you just need to indicate care guides used and sign to confirm care given. However, if there are variations from the planned care, you need to record the variation and action taken on the variation record.

Where do we keep a unified record? The ideal answer is to keep the record with the patient. However, this requires a culture change by everyone, and staff need to debate issues such as confidentiality, access and security. When it comes to filing the record in the case notes, a unified record creates problems if the case notes are filed by profession rather than in chronological order.

Why do we need ICPs and where do they fit in? ICPs are a good idea for patients undergoing straightforward investigations or procedures. However, when care gets complex, for example a stroke patient with diabetes and chest pain, ICPs lack flexibility. A UPR can cope with this situation by using care guides, protocols and mini-plans, depending on the needs of the patient.

Why don't we wait for the EPR to do this for us? EPR clinical documentation will not be available until at least 2005. This gives us time to alter our mindset to accommodate a modern approach to clinical record keeping, including getting used to the language and making records concise and timely.

How can it be an individual record if it's standardised? The UPR is more flexible than an ICP because, as well as accentuating what's special about the patient using documentation by exception, it uses care guides based on individual need.

How do we know who's accountable when recording is done by dots? Who is accountable for the dots recorded on an observation chart? Charts are records too and most are annotated by dots. The registered nurse signs off the GPP to show that she has supervised all care/treatment and is accountable for the care that has been given for that shift. So, even if charts have been initialled by other members of the team, the registered nurse verifies the care by his or her signature.

Where do we record an incident? You should follow normal trust procedure for incident reporting and record the incident as a variation to normal care.

Where do we record complicated discharge? We have struggled with this problem since the beginning of the changes to record keeping. A complete solution may not be possible on paper, so we may need to wait for EPR. An interim solution is a unified weekly communication sheet for complex discharge planning, which is used as the basis for discharge planning meetings.

If we decide to make our record patient-held whilst the patient is in hospital, how do we handle sensitive issues? In our experience, if you record the facts then there is no harm in the patient reading them. In the case of recording preliminary diagnoses, an open and honest approach with the patient is necessary to prevent misunderstandings. If you need to record abusive behaviour of a patient or their family, as long as the record is factual and objective, there should be no problems.

If the record is at the patient's bedside, how do we prevent others reading it? In a typical ward, the notes trolley is central, and open to access by whoever is passing. Records at the bedside are generally protected by the patient. However, if the patient is not capable of this, common sense must prevail. A bedside drawer is a good place to store records out of sight.

8

Toolkit for the development of a unified patient record

This chapter gives practical advice about carrying out a project, based on our four years' experience with the Weston project. Preparation for the project should include exercises such as a SWOT and force field analysis, along with a thorough literature review. Prince project management is the recommended NHS methodology for large projects. Its principles are ideal to help with planning and documenting projects. For more details, go to www.prince2.com.

How to start the process of change

1 Ensure that board level support has been agreed for the project.
2 Arrange an introductory session, inviting all clinicians.
3 Set the context with a presentation.
4 Facilitate discussion – what we think of the current record and what we think will happen in the future, the EPR, where data collection meets recording of care.
5 Agree some objectives the project group need to achieve:

- patient as focus of care (bringing the service to the patient, rather than expecting them to fit in with the service), meaning that care/service is provided in the most appropriate form, by the most appropriate individual, and in the most effective fashion, i.e. integrated care
- a means by which new practices and high standards are structurally incorporated into patient management, so that they will remain so (not just a paper exercise, but a lasting culture change)
- a means by which routine care can be monitored to ensure consistent best practice, and exceptions to the routine can be studied for their 'deviation' from the norm and to inform routine practice (a dynamic process).

6 Decide within the group who should be involved in the change and what the ground rules should be.
7 Identify a project team, including a project lead.
8 Initiate planning, timings, etc.
9 Set date for start of activity and next meeting.

How to establish a baseline

Look at existing audit results or, if none exist, carry out audit of structure and clinical content of existing records, using the group to audit and interpret results. Use existing audit criteria such as:

1 NMC *Guidelines for Records and Record-keeping*[1]
2 King's Fund *Documentation Audit Tool*[2]
3 tools from *Setting the Records Straight*[3]
4 benchmark current practice using the record-keeping section in the Department of Health *The Essence of Care* benchmarking toolkit.[4]

How to develop a framework for collecting information

- Carry out process mapping of patient journeys and the resulting collection of clinical information.
- Use computer terminology such as 'report' instead of letter, version numbers, codes for professions, etc., to familiarise staff with the language.

- Consider incorporating data collection traditionally carried out as a separate exercise, for example national data returns such as MINAP (Myocardial Infarction National Audit Programme).
- Does the resulting booklet need to be stapled to avoid the pages becoming mixed up and for easier storage?
- Aids to navigation of a new record include an index of pages, document numbering and version control.
- Put together a basic first draft and pilot it, not waiting until it's perfect.

How to use existing integrated care pathways

Ask yourself the following questions:

- Have you already developed pathways?
- Consider the success of your approach – has it achieved information-based changes to practice?
- Has it become easier to collect data and monitor practice?
- Are your pathways standardised, clearly written and unambiguous?
- Is there the potential to use pieces of pathways to create a generic record that covers all patients?

Tip: use your existing pathway groups to design, implement and evaluate a new unified record.

How to develop evidence-based care guides

- Do you have a system for integrating evidence into practice, which is accessible at ward/department level by all who contribute to care? If not, then start from scratch with multiprofessional groups, each of which can investigate a topic of their choice.
- Topics may be chosen from personal interest, from patient-related incidents or complaints. For example, a multidisciplinary care guide for the care of a fine bore nasogastric tube was created in response to an incident involving nasogastric feeding.
- Existing guidelines can form the basis of care guides and should do so, if they exist. For example, the care guide for pressure ulcer prevention incorporates the Waterlow score and evidence about pressure-relieving equipment.
- Each care guide must have an author, date of production and date of review.

- Put a storage mechanism in each ward area – could be a folder (A5 on the nurses' station is best), the intranet, pocket files for each clinician or a combination of all three. Make sure the storage mechanism is the same everywhere, to help staff use the care guides whichever ward they work on.
- All staff are individually responsible for ensuring they have read the care guides before use. This accountability is necessary to ensure that when they sign to say they have actioned a care guide, they have acknowledged its contents. This should be pointed out during training.

How to make arrangements to use the Gloucester Patient Profile

Get permission from the clinical governance department at Gloucester-shire Royal Infirmary to use the GPP. A sample copy can be found at www.avon.nhs.uk/imtconsortium/publications but this is unsuitable for printing in large numbers.

Tip: do not photocopy the GPP – it breaks copyright and costs a fortune in coloured ink!

How to do a pilot, and learn from it

Things to consider prior to the start of the pilot include the following.

- Choose a pilot site carefully – identify champions and good leadership in the area of the pilot.
- Decide upon the details of the pilot – length of time, methods of evaluation, review dates and criteria for making changes.
- Ensure that clinicians from the pilot site are involved in designing the record and arranging the pilot.
- Publicise the pilot within the ward team and in other areas – choose a start date and stick to it. **Tip:** put posters in staff toilets to ensure that everyone reads them!
- Ensure that all staff receive training, including ward clerks, night staff and all disciplines, including dietitians, specialist nurses, etc.

- Provide a way of allowing everyone to give written feedback, with a deadline for responses to be included.
- Analyse the feedback, any audit results, and agree resulting changes to the record.

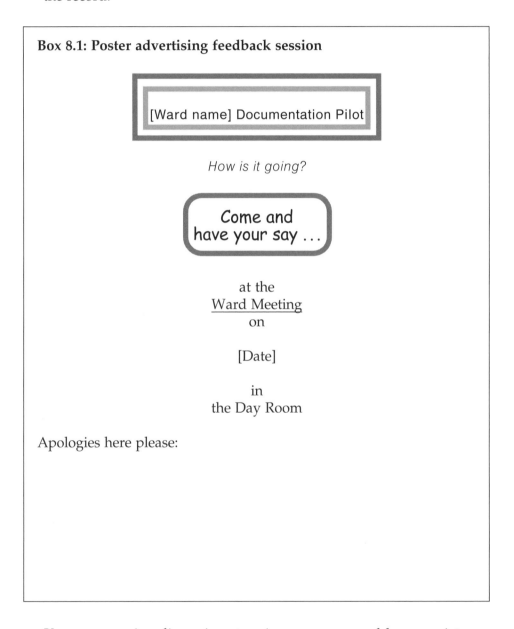

Box 8.1: Poster advertising feedback session

[Ward name] Documentation Pilot

How is it going?

Come and
have your say ...

at the
Ward Meeting
on

[Date]

in
the Day Room

Apologies here please:

- Keep up ongoing discussions to raise awareness and lower resistance. *See* Box 8.2 for an example of written feedback following a discussion with ward sisters about record-keeping issues.

Box 8.2: Extract from a feedback session during a pilot

Advantages and disadvantages of updating the nursing documentation

Problems with care plans

1 Too much repetitive writing.
2 Less time spent with patients.
3 Care plans are often left incomplete.
4 Too much paper.
5 Core care plans are put into documentation and then left blank.
6 Other professions (particularly doctors) find them hard to navigate.

Advantages with care plans

1 Nurses are used to writing them.
2 Systems are already in place for obtaining, storing and using them.

Problems with new patient record

1 Documenting by exception means that routine care is signed for by outcome (patient is free from sore areas, etc.) so detailed care is not actually written down every time, but relies on pre-written guidelines.
2 Much education is needed to ensure everyone knows how to use it.
3 It is uncertain whether a complaint can be answered better with the new patient record than with the old nursing documentation.

Advantages with new patient record

1 The format is the same as integrated care pathways – all professions use this for stroke and total hip replacement so far.
2 There is better representation of trends in the patient's condition using the GPP.
3 The system will change the way nurses record care – this needs to be prepared for the electronic patient record.

But ...
• Neither system can solve the problem of dodgy quality recording of care.
• Electronic systems rely on the use of guidelines.
• There is no point in changing the documentation unless we can move it forward.
• Recording every aspect of the patient's care every time it happens is unrealistic (audit has shown this many times).
• To focus too much on recording every aspect of complex care will ensure that the new patient record is merely the Roper model by another name.
• To record *variations* from the care detailed in guidelines is the only way of sifting what is special about the patient – good risk management practice.

- Evaluate the pilot as you go along, keeping a record of all audit activity.
- Review all audit results and verbal/written feedback at a pre-arranged review meeting.
- Incorporate feedback into improved design.

How to prepare for rollout

1 Obtain board level ratification of new policies to reflect the changes to practice, including a sound policy that supports the use of care guides.
2 Create guidelines and circulate to ward clerks to prepare them for the trustwide rollout (*see* Box 8.3).

Box 8.3: Guidelines for ward clerks

New Patient Record
Guidelines for ward clerks

After .... [date], the old nursing records (Kardex and care plans) will no longer be available. Your existing supplies will be replaced with the new patient records currently in use on Birnbeck ward and in the stroke care pathway.

1 How to order new supplies
a) Gloucester Patient Profile – phone stores and order them by name. When the current supply runs out (in about six months) you will be issued with a WSM order number for the next batch.
b) Front Page – called Doc 1. Will come up with the patient from A&E, along with the first GPP. The front page is available from the print room if needed for patients who do not come through A&E.
c) Other Pages:

Index	Doc 2
Home Life Assessment	Doc 3
Variation Record	Doc 4
Blank Complex Care Plan	Doc 5
Daily Record of Care	Doc 6
Patient's Page	Doc 7
Nursing Guidelines	Doc 8

These can be collected from the print room using the usual order form (an updated version).

---

2 How to file the new records
The records should be filed in the back of the notes, in the same order as the Doc numbers (for example, front page first – Doc 1; all daily record sheets together – Doc 6 – in date order).

Training in the way the new nursing records are used is available every afternoon in August from 2.30 to 3pm in Birnbeck ward's day room. Please feel free to go and find out how they work.

3 Distribute sample sets of the new record to the wards, along with an explanation of what they are (*see* Box 8.4).

Box 8.4: Label for sample sets of records

Sample set of new patient records

To replace Kardex/care plans

from [date]

Go to Birnbeck ward at 2.30 any afternoon in August to receive training

---

4 Implement trustwide education, using a variety of strategies such as posters, on-the-job training and flexible training sessions given by those involved in the pilot.
    Tip: create a sticker to give to those who attend (*see* Box 8.5).

Box 8.5: Example of a sticker

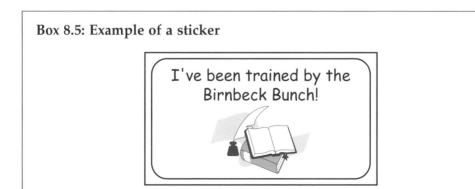

5   Display posters in all clinical areas (*see* Figure 8.1).

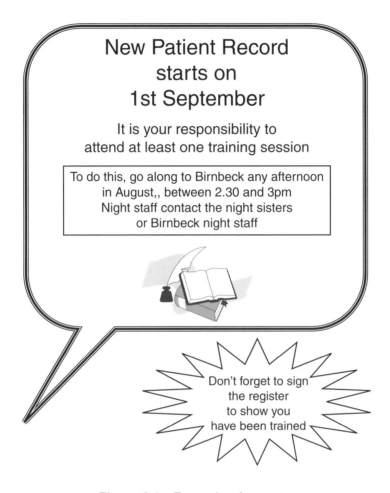

Figure 8.1   Example of a poster

6   Make sure plenty of guidance is available to give people information about the change.
7   Assemble a training pack to be included in the care guides folder, as well as being used to train all staff. Include a completed copy of the patient record and Gloucester Patient Profile, as well as the NMC *Guidelines for Records and Record-keeping*.[1]

Box 8.6: Weston Area Health Trust care guides

What are they?

Care guides are trustwide guidelines for nursing and other care. They are evidence-based and exist to provide a consistent approach to every aspect of care given locally. As *guides*, they should complement but not replace professional judgement, especially at times when alternative care needs to be given. This is made clearer in the mouthcare example below.

Where have they come from?

Much of the care we give has been taught during our training and we keep to that practice through thick and thin! However, things change – using research findings to update practice is now commonplace. Care guides have been created in this way by nurses looking at areas of practice and applying the best evidence. Core care plans were early versions of this, and will often form the basis of new up-to-date practices. The process is never-ending, and is part of clinical governance. The next step in the process is to make care guides multidisciplinary. The stroke pathway is a good example of this.

Where do they fit in?

The new patient record is designed to be concise, prevent duplication and allow nurses to spend more time with the patient. To do this, the method used is recording by exception. This means that normal everyday care is signed off as having been given, but elements of how it is given are not explicit within the record. Care guides provide the detail of care given.

What is my responsibility?

You are accountable for the care you give. Because you are not recording every aspect of that care, you need to be able to demonstrate that you know and adhere to the care guides. When you sign to say that, for example, 'the patient has had mouthcare', you must be satisfied that you have followed the trust care guide for mouthcare. If you haven't followed the care guide, you must record the reason on the variation record and the alternative action taken – recording by exception.

Box 8.7: The Gloucester Patient Profile (GPP)

What is it?

The GPP was developed by staff in the stroke unit at Gloucestershire Royal Infirmary. It is based on the Barthel functional assessment. It is now used across all the Gloucester trusts as part of their patient records. It has been tested and refined whilst in use on Birnbeck ward and has recently been introduced via the stroke integrated care pathway.

What is it for?

It allows complete recording of the patient's condition in a format similar to an observation chart. This means that changes in condition can be seen at a glance by whichever profession looks at the chart.

Why is it so complicated?

It looks complicated, but once you get used to it, it takes less than a minute to complete each column. It reduces the amount of handwriting (free text) needed. It does not, however, replace the need for a record of care; it merely provides a record of condition to complement it.

What are the colours for?

The colours resemble traffic lights. They can be used as an indication of the patient's condition:

- Red — dependent.
- Yellow — less dependent.
- Green — independent.

The sections in the GPP can be viewed separately, or can be totalled and form a colour-based dependency scoring system. This means that when the GPP is in full use, there will be a consistent way across the trust of understanding dependency levels.

How is it used?

Each patient has a GPP when they are first admitted. On the left hand side are columns labelled P and A. These are to record the patient's 'previous' condition and 'actual' condition. This replaces the Roper assessment of activities of daily living with something more precise and complete.
The GPP is completed once a shift – Birnbeck ward took part in the pilot study and found it best to complete it on drug rounds.

RGNs mark the boxes *with a dot* and sign off the record at the bottom of the last page.
Unqualified nurses *initial* the boxes and sign their names on the last page – in this case, a trained nurse still has to sign the last page to confirm that this is indeed the condition of the patient.

Each GPP lasts a week.

How does the GPP improve things for the patient?

1   The first question on the GPP is 'are you feeling better, the same or worse?' Because you are asking this question three times a day, and recording the answer, you are ensuring that you listen to the patient and show that their opinion is important.
2   Because the recording is concise, you will find that you can spend less time on paperwork overall and more time with patients.
3   Communication is improved because all professions can see the condition of the patient at a glance – the GPP is kept at the end of the bed.

How does it improve things for us?

The last page of the GPP includes mobility risk and Waterlow assessments. These are incorporated into the document, so that it is easier to repeat and record them as per trust policy. The pressure sore 'yes/no' column provides a way of collecting information about pressure sores automatically, rather than trying to remember the last three months' figures when the ward is asked for them. The GPP works in conjunction with the new patient record, particularly the daily care record. This means that there is less duplication of writing and recording of care.

The electronic patient record (EPR) will soon be with us. The change in recording style that the GPP brings will ensure that we are more ready to take on the EPR when it arrives.

What if I have other questions?

Staff on Birnbeck ward have been using the GPP for eight months and will be pleased to answer any questions you may have.

Ensure trustwide guidelines for use of the record are available, as in the examples in Box 8.8.

Box 8.8: General guidelines for use of the patient record

WESTON AREA HEALTH NHS TRUST
(Guidelines to support the record-keeping policy)

The patient record is designed to allow multi-professions to record care in a precise and accurate format. The assessment tool calculates the patient's functional ability and presents it in a standardised format. This allows easy reference of the patient's condition and trends can be quickly highlighted.

1 The patient record should be used for all inpatients except for where a care pathway exists.
2 The record should be commenced on admission to hospital whether via the accident and emergency department or as a planned admission. The patient should be assessed using the Gloucester Patient Profile (GPP).
3 If patient assessment indicates a need, action should be taken to meet that need. This should be recorded in the record.
4 All sections should be completed.
5 The patient record should be updated at least daily.
6 Changes and additions to the record should be made at the time when the change/addition occurs.
7 At the end of the patient stay, the nurse discharging the patient should check that the patient record is complete, including discharge details, before the record is filed in the patient's notes.

Further reading
● Department of Health (2001) *Essence of Care*. DoH, London.
● Department of Health (1999) *For the Record: managing records in NHS trusts and health authorities*. Health Service Circular, 1999/053. DoH, London.

Box 8.9: General guidelines for use of the Gloucester Patient Profile

WESTON AREA HEALTH NHS TRUST
(Guidelines to support the record-keeping policy)

The Gloucester Patient Profile is a double-sided two page patient assessment, the core of which is based on the Barthel Index. The document enables plotting of a patient's condition over seven days. This is a functional assessment tool and each section of the assessment has three statements about the patient. The statements are colour-coded green ▨ , amber ▨ or red ▨ . Green indicates 'independence' in a function, amber indicates 'requires assistance' and red indicates that the patient is 'dependent'.

This allows a thorough assessment of the patient and concise collection of clinical information.

1 Registered nurses record information on the GPP by dotting with a black pen in each statement. All other staff initial each section. The registered nurse supervising the patient's care for each shift must sign on the back page. All other staff must identify their initials once in the box provided on the back page.

2 On admission, the patient should be assessed by a registered nurse using the P and A column on the left side of the chart. The P is the patient's previous ability when fit and well and the A is the patient's actual ability on admission.

3 Any notes about a function can be made on page 3. The notes should be concise and can be linked to any function they affect. For example, a patient with back pain could find that notes will apply to more than one function, e.g. pain, mobility, sitting, standing, moving in bed, etc. The number of the note should be put in all applicable boxes by the function.

4 Patients should have a full assessment once a day. This should be done in the morning to allow any changes to be addressed during the day. Consecutive staff during the evening or night must sign to say that they agree with the previous assessment. If the patient's condition changes during the shift they should be reassessed and a record made.

5 When a patient is assessed as being in a red or amber zone they should have a care guide or complex care plan in use to address this.

6 Other assessments included in the GPP are the Waterlow and mobility risk assessment. The patients' Waterlow should be assessed every third day or when there is a material change in

their condition. A pressure area care guide should be used for all patients with a Waterlow of above 10; where the patients have existing pressure damage they should have a complex care plan. When patients are assessed as category B or C in mobility they should have a complex mobility risk assessment completed.

7 It is important that the nurse notes on admission whether the patient has any existing pressure damage. This should be reviewed at least daily and recorded on the back page of the GPP.

8 The type of mattress used for the patient should be recorded on the back of the GPP.

9 All patients should have their GPP assessments completed daily, unless there has been a local agreement to reduce or increase frequency.

Further reading

- Allen D (1998) Record-keeping and routine practice: the view from the wards. *J Adv Nurs*.
- UKCC (1998) *Guidelines for Records and Record Keeping*. UKCC, London.
- Department of Health (1999) *For the Record: managing records in NHS trusts and health authorities*. DoH, London.

8 Audit/monitor implementation.

Things to expect during the project

Disruption is inevitable and, as with any major change in practice, time is needed to embed the new system and achieve high quality record-keeping practices. The following difficulties are to be expected and should be addressed as they arise.

- Discomfort at losing the requirement to write everything down. Although this was never achieved in practice, nurses in particular were used to the principle. Care guides make writing everything down unnecessary by making aspects of care implicit within the new way of recording.
- Impact of change. Professionals need to absorb the new way of recording, but this means that, for a while, a certain amount of chaos

in record-keeping habits exists. Problems such as forgetting to write the patient's name on each page or filing the record in the wrong order existed in the old documentation but will be temporarily accentuated.

- Those who do not see the benefits of the new way of recording will grumble, which creates a disabling atmosphere for those trying to adapt to the change. The documentation link group understand the benefits and will be a positive influence.
- Time and staff constraints mean that training needs will never be met in full. Ad hoc training and cascade learning should be employed, and a web-based solution to help with ongoing training needs would help. Training should never be underestimated, but always is!

How to maintain the momentum of the project

1 Be prepared for:

- lack of time for meetings, along with difficulty in finding a day and time suitable for each profession
- lack of attendance at meetings, whilst acknowledging that small meetings are often the most productive
- cultural differences between the professions, which warrant the need for much face-to-face discussion and learning of each other's roles. Barriers to this include the amount and complexity of nursing documentation – other professions find it difficult to read information pertinent to them
- discussion about the issue of consent, both for procedures that already use a 'consent form' and for those that currently have informal consent, such as thrombolysis, or CT scan. At what point in the process consent is given, the amount of time the patient is given to absorb any information, and the way it is presented are also areas for discussion
- the need for development of patient information alongside the documentation, bringing forth the problem of accurately assessing what is currently available and finding valid and reliable tools to test new leaflets; also patient involvement in the writing and testing of information
- practical problems, such as the improvement of working practices to meet nationally agreed guidelines, hampered by practical issues such as availability of equipment and services
- cultural change, such as where to keep the documents, and how to change nursing handover to avoid the use of the 'Kardex'.

2 Benchmark effectiveness of care.
3 Control versions and update the record.
4 Derive management information from clinical information.

How to provide ongoing training

1 Decide changes needed to current training programmes, such as continuing education on both how to use the new patient record, and principles of good record keeping.
2 Use link clinicians to give training.
3 Inclusion of training in the induction of all new staff, including return-to-practice nurses, adaptation nurses, NVQ students and cadets.
4 Produce a newsletter, or ensure regular inclusion in trustwide publications.

This toolkit consists of strategies we have tried that have worked. However, do expand upon these and be creative in your approach. In our experience, one of the most important aspects of a project such as this is to listen to staff and ensure their ideas are incorporated.

Finally . . .

Tip: a touch of humour always helps.

References

1   Nursing and Midwifery Council (2002) *Guidelines for Records and Record-keeping*. NMC, London.
2   King's Fund (1995) *Documentation Audit Tool*. King's Fund, London.
3   Audit Commission (1997) *Setting the Records Straight*. HMSO, London.
4   Department of Health (2001) *The Essence of Care: patient-focused benchmarking for healthcare practitioners*. DoH, London. www.doh.gov.uk/essenceofcare

9

Example of a unified patient record

Gloucester Patient Profile

Weston Area Health Trust Patient Record

- Home life assessment
- Discharge planning checklist
- Complex mobility risk assessment
- Variation record
- Plan of complex care
- Daily record of care
- Weekly record of care
- Patient's page

Care guides
- Care guide for bowel preparation
- Care guide for use of central lines
- Care guide for a blocked central line
- Care guide for fine bore nasogastric feeds
- Care guide for hypoglycemia

Unified specialist assessments and records
- Tissue viability record
- Critical care record

THE GLOUCESTER PATIENT PROFILE	NAME						D.O.B.		GO		W/C	

P	A		M	E	N	M	E	N	M	E	N	M	E	N	M	E	N	M	E	N	M	E	N	M	E	N

WELLBEING — See Note

		2	Patient feels general condition is improving
		1	Patient feels general condition is unchanged
		0	Patient feels general condition is worsening

COMMUNICATION — See Note

		3	Can communicate verbally
		2	Limited verbal communication
		2	Communicates by writing
		1	Uses only gestures/communication aids
		0	Unable to communicate

COMPREHENSION — See Note

		3	Understands complex sequences/sentences
		2	Understands simple sequences/sentences
		1	Single word comprehension
		0	No apparent comprehension

SPEECH — See Note

		3	Speech normal
		2	Variable slurred speech
		1	Constant slurred speech
		0	Unable to speak

ORIENTATION — See Note

		2	Appears fully alert and orientated
		1	Appears mildly confused/disorientated
		0	Severe confusion and/or disorientation

MEMORY — See Note

		2	Short and long term recall
		1	Variable short and/or long term recall
		0	Constant short and/or long term loss

PLANNED ACTIVITY — See Note

		3	Mobile as able
		2	Restricted mobility
		1	Chair rest
		0	Bed rest

SITTING — See Note

		2	Able to sit unsupported
		1	Able to sit with assistance/positioning
		0	Unable to sit

STANDING — See Note

		2	Independent
		1	Requires assistance
		0	Unable to stand

MOVEMENT IN BED — See Note

		2	Independent
		1	Requires assistance
		0	Unable to move

PAIN — See Note

		2	No pain
		1	Pain controlled by analgesia
		0	Episodes of uncontrolled pain

P	A		M	E	N	M	E	N	M	E	N	M	E	N	M	E	N	M	E	N	M	E	N
		BARTHEL ADL INDEX (ADAPTED)																					
		BLADDER See Note																					
	2	Continent																					
	1	Catheter or sheath																					
	0	Incontinent																					
		Passed urine																					
		BOWELS See Note																					
	2	Continent																					
	1	Oral aperient																					
	0	Enema or suppository																					
	0	Incontinent																					
		Bowels opened																					
		TOILET See Note																					
	2	Independent																					
	1	Requires help																					
	0	Dependent																					
		MOBILITY See Note																					
	3	Independent																					
	2	Independent with supervision																					
	2	Assistance from one person																					
	1	Assistance from two or more people																					
	0	Immobile																					
		TRANSFERS See Note																					
	3	Independent																					
	2	Requires supervision																					
	1	Requires assistance																					
	0	Dependent																					
		STAIRS See Note																					
	2	Independent																					
	1	Requires assistance																					
	0	Unable to climb or descend stairs																					
		GROOMING See Note																					
	1	Independent																					
	0	Manages upper body – lower with assistance																					
	0	Dependent																					
		BATHING See Note																					
	1	Independent																					
	0	Requires supervision																					
	0	Requires assistance																					
	0	Dependent																					
		DRESSING See Note																					
	2	Independent																					
	1	Manages upper – lower with assistance																					
	1	Upper with assistance – dependent for lower																					
	0	Dependent																					
		FEEDING See Note																					
	2	Independent																					
	1	Requires help cutting up food – feeds self																					
	1	Requires assistance or supervision																					
	0	Unable to feed self – requires feeding																					
		TOTALS																					

P	A				M	E	N	M	E	N	M	E	N	M	E	N	M	E	N	M	E	N	M	E	N	M	E	N
AIRWAY			See Note																									
		2	Able to maintain own airway																									
		1	Maintains own airway – requires observation																									
		1	Requires assistance to maintain airway																									
		0	Unable to maintain airway																									
SHORT OF BREATH			See Note																									
		2	No abnormality with ordinary activity																									
		2	SOB with some activity (e.g. stairs)																									
		1	SOB walking on flat surfaces																									
		1	SOB with mild exertion (washing/dressing)																									
		0	SOB at rest and on talking																									
BREATHING			See Note																									
		2	Breathes normally – without assistance																									
		1	Change to normal pattern (observation)																									
		1	Change to normal pattern (intervention)																									
		0	Unable to breathe without assistance																									
TYPE OF DIET			See Note																									
		2	Normal diet																									
		2	Modified diet																									
		1	Fluids only																									
		0	Nil by mouth																									
ROUTE OF DIET			See Note																									
		2	Oral																									
		1	Tube (state type)																									
		0	Intravenous																									
APPETITE			See Note																									
		2	Full appetite																									
		1	Changed appetite																									
		0	Not eating																									
GUT FUNCTION			See Note																									
		2	Normal																									
		1	Changed gut function																									
		0	No gut function																									
SWALLOWING			See Note																									
		2	Eats and drinks normally																									
		1	Drinks normally, modified diet																									
		1	Sips fluids, modified diet																									
		0	Unable to swallow, nil by mouth																									
SLEEP			See Note																									
		2	Undisturbed sleep																									
		2	Disturbed sleep (satisfactory to patient)																									
		1	Disturbed sleep (unsatisfactory to patient)																									
		0	Unable to sleep																									

No	Date	Note	Entry by:	Discontinued by:	Date
1					
2					
3					
4					
5					
6					
7					
8					

MOBILITY RISK ASSESSMENT

Category A: Patient is able to fully mobilise
Category B: Patient needs verbal encouragement from staff/possible use of simple aids to mobilise themselves in this environment
Category C: Patient needs manual help from staff/aids and/or hoist equipment to mobilise in this environment
Manual Handling Guidelines
Please complete Complex Mobility Risk Assessment form if the patient is in **Risk Category C** in any activity
Complete a plan on the form each time the patient's ability changes

P	A	MOBILITY RISK ASSESSMENT	M	E	N	M	E	N	M	E	N	M	E	N	M	E	N	M	E	N	M	E	N
		Category A:																					
		Category B:																					
		Category C:																					
Complex Mobility Risk Assessment up-to-date? (Y/N)																							

WATERLOW PRESSURE SORE RISK

Build/weight for height. Average 0 Above average 1 Well above average 2 Below average 3	
Continence. Complete/catheter 0 Occ. incontinence 1 Catheter/inco. of faeces 2 Doubly incontinent 3	
Appetite. Average 0 Poor 1 NG tube/fluids only 2 NBM/anorexic 3	
Mobility. Fully 0 Restless/fidgety 1 Apathetic 2 Restricted 3 Inert/traction 4 Chairbound 5	
Sex/Age. Male 1 Female 2. 14–49 = 1 50–64 = 2 65–74 = 3 75–80 = 4 81+ = 5	
Skin type/risk areas. Healthy 0 Tissue paper 1 Dry 1 Clammy 1 Oedema 1 Discoloured 2 Broken 3	
Tissue malnutrition. Smoking 1 Anaemia 2 Per. Vasc. Disease 5 Card. Failure 5 Term Cachexia 8	
Neurological deficit. e.g. Diabetes, MS, CVA, Motor/Sensory, Paraplegia 4–6	
Major surgery. Orthopaedic below waist – spinal 5 On table > 2 hours 5	
Medication. Steroids, Cytotoxics, High dose anti-flammatory 4	
TOTAL	
Pressure sore present (Y = yes N = no)	

TYPE OF MATTRESS (ENTER CODE IN BOX)

1	
2	
TIME	
SIGNATURES	

	Initials	Signature	Name (print)	Grade		Initials	Signature	Name (print)	Grade
1					4				
2					5				
3					6				

(*See* page 89 for key to assessing patient's condition.)

WESTON AREA HEALTH TRUST
PATIENT RECORD

Unit no. . . . .

Surname (Mr/Mrs/Ms/Miss). . . . .

Forename(s). . . . .

Patient address . . . .

. . . .

. . . .

DOB. . . . .

Temp. address. . . . .

. . . .

. . . .

Religion . . . .

Occupation . . . .

Ethnic origin . . . .

Presenting problem

Diagnosis/operation

Resus. status

Signature . . . .

Date. . . . .

Nursing team

Consultant. . . . .

Other healthcare professionals

. . . .

Date and time of admission

. . . .

Ward . . . .

Admitted from . . . .

Date transferred . . . .

Transfer ward . . . .

First contact

Name. . . . .

Relationship. . . . .

Address . . . .

. . . .

. . . .

Tel. no. (day) . . . .

Tel. no. (night). . . . .

Aware of admission? Y/N

Contact day or night? Y/N

Other contact

Name. . . . .

Relationship. . . . .

Address . . . .

. . . .

Tel. no. (day) . . . .

Tel. no. (night) . . . .

GP name . . . .

Address . . . .

Tel. no. . . . .

Property disclaimer signed in A&E?

Yes/No. If no, use property book

Discl. no. . . . .

Mental health details

Physical description

Eye colour . . . .

Hair colour . . . .

Build: slight/medium/stocky/large

Distinguishing features . . . .

. . . .

Past nursing and medical history (to include any appointments which may need cancelling) and significant life events

---

Height	Weight	Medicines retained by ward? Y/N

Urinalysis

Allergies?

A&E Section

Tick all applicable boxes below	Initials
Normal medications **Medicines brought in with patient (Y/N)** **Please list**	
Nil by mouth **Since _ _ _ _ _ hrs**	
Oxygen given **If 'Yes' state percentage**	
Fluids commenced **State site of cannula** IV S/C **State size of cannula**	
Catheterised Urinary sheath **If catheterised: size and batch number:**	
Bloods taken FBC INR Others – please state: *Results to be recorded in notes* ESR U&Es	
Investigations undertaken Chest X-Ray Others – please state: ECG Others	

Baseline observations done? (see observation chart)

Temp	Pulse	Resps.	ECG	Sats	BP	Pupils
BM mmol/L	Urinalysis	Waterlow score	GCS Eye **/4** Motor **/6** Verbal **/5** Neurological chart started Y/N *(delete)* Time interval:			

Information given to patient and/or relatives

A/E plan

A/E nurse _ _ _ _ _ _ _ _ _ _ _ _ Date _ _ _

HOME LIFE ASSESSMENT

Ward:

Date:

	Hospital no:
Name:	
DoB:	Affix label here

ACCOMMODATION – please delete where appropriate

Type of accommodation

House/bungalow ☐

Flat – ground floor/other ☐

Ownership of accommodation

Owned/rented – local authority/private
landlord/housing association ☐

Residential home/nursing home ☐

Warden controlled ☐

Other (please state) ☐

Stairs/stair lift/steps leading up to entrance of accommodation

Internal ☐   External ☐

Yes ☐   No ☐   Yes ☐   No ☐

If Yes, state how many

Toilet   Upstairs ☐   Downstairs ☐   Both ☐

Bathroom   Upstairs ☐   Downstairs ☐   Both ☐
              Bath ☐   Shower ☐

Bedroom   Upstairs ☐   Downstairs ☐   Both ☐

Is there a room to sleep downstairs?   Yes/No

Is the patient in receipt of any benefits? Yes/No

CARE/SUPPORT/SOCIAL NETWORK

Lives alone? Yes/No
If No, with whom?

Tel. no.   Relationship

Tel. no.   Relationship

Contact telephone number:

Carer details (if different)

Care giver to other(s)?   Yes/No
If Yes, to whom?

Health/social service support received prior to admission? Yes/No
If Yes, tick relevant boxes

Meals on wheels ☐   Day centre care ☐

Home care ☐   District nurse ☐

CPN ☐   Social worker ☐

Other ☐

If other, please specify

Contact details

Name

Tel. no.

Telephone/carelink/alarm? Yes/No

Appointments cancelled?   Yes/No
If Yes, please specify

Leisure/occupation/hobbies

Car owner/driver ☐   Orange badge holder? ☐   Clubs, hobbies etc. ☐

Other details not covered above

Signature of assessor(s):

DISCHARGE PLANNING CHECKLIST

Proposed date of discharge: **Actual date of discharge:**

Named nurse/key worker to complete.

Team members aware of discharge planning
Initial and date boxes when staff have been notified.

Team members	
Named nurse	
Consultant	
Physiotherapist	
Occupational therapist	
Relatives/carers/friends	
Social worker	
District nurse	
Dietitian (if involved)	

Where is the patient going on discharge?

OT visit needed before discharge? Yes/No
Initial and date boxes

If yes, patient has: clothes on ward	
key for home on ward	
Relative/carer/friend is aware	
Social worker is aware	
District nurse is aware	
Home visit page commenced	

Date and time of first home visit

Transport arranged for home visit? Yes/No

If yes, state mode of transport arranged

Details of discharge

	Yes	No
Transport required?		
If yes, transport booked?		
am/pm		
If yes, state mode of transport arranged		
Discharge drugs required?		
If yes, discharge drugs obtained		
If yes, discharge drugs explained		
Explained to person other than patient?		
Name		
Patient's own property/drugs returned?		
Discharge letters/certificates		
Discharge letter printed (x3)		
Transfer letter to district nurse		
Transfer letter to resi/nursing home?		
Transfer letter to other hospital?		
Medical/DSS certificate given		
Outpatient appointment booked		
Written details given to: patient		
other relative/carer		
Transport arranged for appointment		
If yes, state mode of transport arranged		
Variations, and other action taken		

COMPLEX MOBILITY RISK ASSESSMENT

This patient's mobility has been assessed for risk and should therefore mobilise as shown below.

Name: **Unit no:**

Task	Date with signature and recommended equipment			
Turn to right in bed				
Turn to left in bed				
Up and down bed				
Lying to sitting				
Sitting to standing				
Transfer bed to chair/wheelchair				
Transfer on/off toilet/commode				
Wheelchair mobility				
Walking				
On/off floor	Hoist	Hoist	Hoist	Hoist

KEY
0 = Independent	ZF	= Zimmer frame
1 = Help of 1	WZF	= Wheeled zimmer frame
2 = Help of 2	W/S	= Walking stick
3 = Help of 3	Tx Board	= Transfer board
x = Inappropriate	Multiglide	

This information should be updated if any of the circumstances change.

VARIATION RECORD

Ward:

Hospital no:
Name:
DoB: Affix label here

Profession: D=doctor, N=nurse, OT=Occupational therapist, DT=Dietitian, PH=Physiotherapist, SW=Social worker, SLT=Speech and language therapist, SPEC=Specialist nurse

Date and time	Profession (enter code)	Variation report	Signature

PLAN OF COMPLEX CARE

Ward:

Date plan commenced:

Hospital no:

Name:

DoB: Affix label here

Planned care/guidelines and action taken

Signature of nurse planning care   ....

Date and signature of each update   ....

          ....

          ....

          ....

          ....

DAILY RECORD OF CARE

Ward:

Date:

	Hospital no:
Name:	
DoB:	Affix label here

Please initial appropriate box as each item is considered and action completed

Guidelines to be followed/care to be given

	M	E	N		M	E	N
Assistance with hygiene (see GPP)				**Patient/carer communication**			
Patient has had: bath/shower/assisted wash/shave				Psychological wellbeing			
mouthcare/hair washed				Patient feels supported and well-informed			
				Relatives have been included			
Pressure area care							
Patient is free from sore areas				**Discharge**			
Preventative plan has changed (Y/N)				Review ongoing care needs			
				Action towards discharge taken			
Mobility							
Last assessment followed				**Complex care plans used today** (please list)			
Assessment modified as required							
Complex care plan in use? (Y/N)							
Intake				**Care guides used today** (please list)			
Cannula in situ Y/N							
Phlebitis score is 0							
Cannula last changed on:							
Intake is acceptable							
All meals have been eaten							

Please write variations from routine care on the variation record.

WEEKLY RECORD OF CARE

Ward: Hospital no: Name: DoB:

Week commencing:	M	E	N	M	E	N	M	E	N	M	E	N	M	E	N	M	E	N	M	E	N
Assistance with hygiene (see GPP)																					
Bath/shower/hair washed																					
Assisted wash																					
Mouthcare																					
Shave																					
Pressure area care																					
Patient is free from sore areas																					
Care guide in use (Y/N)																					
Mobility																					
Last assessment followed																					
Complex care plan in use? (Y/N)																					
Intake																					
No. of cannulae in situ																					
Cannula 1 phlebitis score is 0																					
changed today																					
record site daily																					
Cannula 2 phlebitis score is 0																					
changed today																					
record site daily																					
Intake is acceptable																					
All meals have been eaten																					
Communication																					
Psychological wellbeing																					
Patient feels supported and well-informed																					
Relatives have been included																					
Discharge																					
Review ongoing care needs																					
Action towards discharge taken																					
Complex care plans in use (list below)																					
Other care guides in use (list below)																					

PATIENT'S PAGE

Ward:

Date:

	Hospital no:
Name:	
DoB:	Affix label here

This page is for you to record any comments, or to raise concerns you may have about aspects of your care and the service we provide. Your relatives/carers are also welcome to write on this page. Your care will not be prejudiced by what you write here. You might like to write about:

- any concerns or comments about your treatment or hospital stay
- any questions you would like answered
- any concerns about your discharge from hospital.

Date	Comments

Please feel free to ask for another page if needed.

Care guides

Care guide for bowel preparation

1 Patients requiring bowel prep should receive a full explanation of the procedure.

2 Each dose of bowel prep should be prescribed by the medical team on the once only section of the patient's drug prescription chart.

3 Patients usually receive two doses.

4 Prior to administering the bowel prep ensure the patient knows where the toilet facilities are and has access to a nurse call bell.

5 Following the first dose of bowel prep the patient should consume a bland diet only. This can consist of:
   • steamed, poached or grilled fish
   • clear soup
   • jelly
   • chocolate
   • small portion of potato or white bread.

6 Following the second dose of bowel prep the patient should have clear fluids only.

7 The patient should receive frequent pain assessments during this time. If experiencing pain, the pain guide should be adhered to and medical staff informed immediately.

8 The patient should be advised to consume at least 200ml of oral fluid an hour whilst undergoing bowel prep to avoid dehydration.

9 Medical staff should be informed if the bowel prep is unsuccessful.

10 An entry should be made on the patient's variation page as to the result of the bowel prep.

Author: Uphill ward staff
Date of approval: November 2000
Date of last review: July 2001
Date of next review: July 2002
Version 1.0

Care guide for use of central lines

Hazards of insertion

Sepsis	Air embolism	Pneumothorax
Hydrothorax	Haemorrhage	Haemothorax
Brachial plexus injury	Thoracic duct trauma	Misdirection
Catheter embolism	Thrombosis	Kinking
Cardiac tamponade	Cardiac arrythmias	

1 Following insertion it is the nurses' responsibility to monitor the patient constantly, looking for clinical signs of patient deterioration and informing medical staff if they are concerned.

2 Of paramount importance is the need for a chest X-ray post insertion and the medical staff documenting they are satisfied with the position prior to any fluids or drugs being administered through the line.

3 The nurse should ensure that if the line has more than one lumen, each should be allocated and 'dedicated' or kept for that specific use, thus reducing the risk of inappropriate sampling or inadvertent mixing of drug/fluid administration.

4 The nurse should make sure that any patient who has a central line in situ who then develops a pyrexia or becomes unwell should be examined by a member of the medical staff and the possibility of a central line problem (as outlined above) considered – no matter how long ago the line was put in situ. The medical staff may elect to have the line removed. If the line is removed the nurse must ensure that the tip is ALWAYS sent for MC&S.

5 The nurse must make sure that blood cultures are always considered for any patient with a pyrexia who has any intravenous cannula of any type in situ.

6 The nurse must make sure that no scissors, needles or ridged forceps, such as artery forceps, should ever be used near a central line because of the risk of inadvertently puncturing the line causing a potential air embolism every time the patient inhales.

7 The nurse should ensure that if a puncture in the external portion of the line is suspected the initial treatment would be to kink the line

manually between the perceived puncture and the patient's skin – thus preventing air being inspired by the patient. **This is an emergency and requires emergency treatment**; pull the bell if necessary.

8   The nurse should, with sterile gloves, cover the puncture site with sterile gauze and apply a sterile toothless clamp. Medical staff must be informed urgently and a **sterile patch applied using aseptic technique.** Stores has a sterile repair kit and the bleep holder will be able to access it. If the medical staff feel unable to undertake this procedure then contact Bristol Oncology Centre for advice and probable transfer for the line to be repaired.

Author: Penney Long
Date of approval: June 2001
Date of last review: –
Date of next review: June 2002
Version 1.0

Care guide for a blocked central line

If an occlusion becomes apparent because you cannot *withdraw* a blood sample the following *might* alleviate the situation.

1   Patient coughs, breathes deeply, rolls from side to side, raises his/her arms, performs the valsalva manoeuvre or increases general activity, e.g. walking upstairs. Such actions are not always possible.

2   If none of these actions alleviate the problem or are not a viable option then the following could be attempted.
    • Gentle aspiration, using no smaller than a 10ml syringe.
    • A 0.9% saline flush, or a Hepsal flush, **never** putting pressure on the line to install the flush (*see* unblocking an occluded catheter using a negative pressure approach).

3   At the time of printing there is no definitive advocated answer as to the best solution to dissolve more substantial occlusions – urokinase, streptokinase and TPA are all currently being investigated. In the event of this occlusion not being resolved utilising any of the previous suggestions then it is suggested that the medical officer contact Bristol Oncology Centre and ask what they are currently using to unblock occluded central lines.

4   Please remember that the infusion (of saline, Hepsal, urokinase or whatever) is instilled into the line sufficiently to fill the line but is subsequently withdrawn. It is never infused into the patient.

Author: Penney Long
Date of approval: June 2001
Date of last review: –
Date of next review: June 2002
Version 1.0

Care guide for fine bore nasogastric feeds

1 The decision to pass a fine bore nasogastric tube must be given by a doctor.

2 All tubes should be checked for position following initial insertion and then at least once per shift or if the patient complains of discomfort or feed reflux into the throat. Once checked, the result must be recorded in the patient's records.

3 When placing the tube into the stomach the nurse must observe for signs of coughing or cyanosis, as these may indicate respiratory placement. However, in unconscious patients or those with a poor gag these signs may be absent. The size of tube inserted must be recorded in the patient's records.

4 To check placement of the tube the nurse should first inject 5ml of air down the tube before aspirating. The withdrawn aspirate should be checked against some litmus paper. If blue litmus paper turns pink this indicates an acid reaction. Where possible, pH sensitive strips should be used and the aspirate should read pH 3–4.

5 Patients must be positioned at an angle of no less than 30 degrees whilst receiving the feed.

6 All patients/carers will receive information regarding NG feeding via fine bore tubes.

7 Where possible, consent should be obtained.

8 Feed giving sets must be changed at least every 24hrs; this should be recorded in the nursing records.

9 Flushes should be no more than 50ml of water.

10 Out of hours the emergency feed regime, as written by the dietitian, may be given. The dietitian must see the patient on the next working day.

11 All feed regimes must be prescribed by a dietitian.

12 Where there is concern that the tube is not in place (e.g. patient shows signs of respiratory distress) the feed must be turned off until tube placement is verified by X-ray.

References

- Colagiovanni L (1999) Taking the tube. *Nurs Times*. **95**(21).
- BRI Guidelines.

Author: Deb Thompson
Date of approval: October 2000
Date of last review: July 2001
Date of next review: July 2002
Version 1.0

Care guide for hypoglycemia

1   If the patient can swallow, administer any of the following rapidly absorbed carbohydrates:

- 10g of oral glucose mixed with 30ml of water
- Lucozade 60ml
- Ribena 15ml
- Coca-Cola 80ml
- Fruit juice 50ml
- Sugar – 2 teaspoons
- Sugar lumps – 3
- Dextrosol tabs – 3.

2   Each of these treatments contains 10g of carbohydrate and should be titrated to blood sugar as follows:

- <4mmol   = 10g of carbohydrate
- <2.5mmol   = 20g of carbohydrate
- <1.5mmol   = 30g of carbohydrate.

3   Follow this with a long-acting carbohydrate, e.g. milk and digestive biscuit, or a sandwich, a banana, cereal, or the planned meal.

4   If the patient is unable to swallow because of the hypo, but is conscious, administer one full tube of Hypostop to the gums and massage for one minute. When the patient responds follow this with oral fluids and a long-acting carbohydrate.

5   If the patient is unconscious, contact the doctor who will then administer 50ml of 50% dextrose i.v.

6   If the doctor is not able to attend i.m. glucagon can be given via a verbal message. Only one dose can be given as it removes all the glucose stores from the liver. This should be followed by a meal as soon as possible as the effect can be a little like a hangover. Another dose can be given, if the patient requires it, after several hours when the liver has restocked. This treatment should be avoided where i.v. access can be obtained for i.v. glucose. The blood sugar should be checked 20–30 minutes after treatment.

7   The patient should not experience hyperglycemia if the correct treatment is given.

References

- Hillson R (1996) *Practical Diabetes Care.* Oxford University Press, Oxford.
- ENB 928 (1998) University of West of England, Bristol.

Author: Julie Gould
Date of approval: November 2000
Date of last review: July 2001
Date of next review: July 2001
Version 1.0

Unified specialist assessments and records

TISSUE VIABILITY RECORD

Date:

Name:	Hospital no:
DoB:	Affix label here

Classification of wound
(please tick the appropriate box)

☐ Surgical   ☐ Traumatic   ☐ Leg ulcer
☐ Foot ulcer   ☐ Cellulitis   ☐ Pressure sore

(If pressure sore complete next section)

Other disciplines involved
(please specify)

☐ Dietitian   ☐ Orthopaedic surgeon
☐ Vascular surgeon
☐ Plastic surgeon

Pressure sore details
Grade (1–5 Torrance scale – please specify)
Waterlow score? (please specify)

Damage on admission   ☐ Yes   ☐ No
Referred to tissue viability nurse ☐

Relevant history of pressure sore or contributing factors

Equipment in use
☐ Pressure reducing foam mattress
☐ Pressure relieving cushion
☐ Pressure relieving chair

☐ Alternating pressure mattress
☐ Leg troughs and bed cradle
☐ Other (please specify)

Site of wound (please specify)   **Top (Dorsal)**   **Bottom (Plantar)**

For wound
assessment
see over

Assessment (Please tick unless otherwise specified) Date																			
Nutrition																				
Is the patient eating a high protein diet?																				
Is the patient receiving high protein supplements?																				
Is the patient receiving vitamin therapy?																				
Infection																				
Suspected																				
Confirmed																				
Wound swab taken																				
Wound depth																				
Superficial – red/discoloured																				
Partial thickness – epidermis/dermis																				
Full thickness – subcutaneous																				
Full thickness – extends to bone tendon																				
Wound bed (specify in %)																				
Epithelialising – pink new epidermis																				
Granulating – red, vascular tissue																				
Infected – green																				
Sloughy – yellow																				
Necrotic – black, devitalised																				
Wound measurements (centimetres)																				
Length – longest point																				
Width – widest point																				
Surrounding skin																				
Healthy																				
Tissue paper																				
Clammy/macerated																				
Discoloured																				
Dressings																				
Primary																				
Secondary																				
Bandaging																				
Surrounding skin protected?																				
Number of changes per week																				
Signature																				

CRITICAL CARE ADMISSION HISTORY

ITU or HDU bed requested:

Date: _ _ _ _ _ _ _ _

Time: _ _ _ _ _ _ _ _

Hospital no.
Name:
DoB: Affix label here

Criteria for admission   **Yes/No** *(tick one)*

Assessed by outreach nurse: ☐ ☐   Date: _ _ _ _ _ _ _ _ _   Time: _ _ _ _ _ _ _ _ _

Anaesthetist: ☐ ☐   Date: _ _ _ _ _ _ _ _ _   Time: _ _ _ _ _ _ _ _ _

MRSA admission screen done: ☐ ☐

MRSA positive: ☐ ☐

ITU/HDU admission   Date: _ _ _ _ _ _ _ _ _   Time: _ _ _ _ _ _ _ _ _

Admitted from: _ _ _ _ _ _ _ _ _ _ _ _ _ _ _ _   Prior location: _ _ _ _ _ _ _ _ _ _ _ _

Admission history:

Explanation/action taken: Delay in transfer to ITU: **Yes/No** *(Delete one)*

Valuables: **Storage:**

	Yes	No	With Pt	Pt's locker	Gen office	Other
Glasses						
Teeth						
Watch						
Jewellery						
Cash						
Other						

Nurses's signature: _ _ _ _ _ _ _ _ _ _ _ _ _ _ _ _

TRANSFER INFORMATION FOR PATIENTS WITH TRACHEOSTOMIES

Date transferred to ward: _ _ _ _ _ _ _ _ _ _ _ _ _ _ _ _

Date tracheostomy inserted	
Reason for tracheostomy	
Date of last tracheostomy change	
Type of tracheostomy tube (please state if inner tube present)	
Size	
Type of secretions	
Frequency of suctioning	
Cuff	
Swallow assessment	
Referred to SALT	
Additional information (problems, wound size, dressings, speaking valve, anatomical difficulties, infection, bleeding, size of suction catheters)	
Signature	
Print name	
Date	

CRITICAL CARE INVESTIGATIONS AND RESULTS SUMMARY

Name:	Hospital no:
DoB:	Affix label here

Type of specimen	Date specimen sent	Results summary

CRITICAL CARE DAILY PATIENT RECORD – MEDICAL SECTION

Name:	Hospital no.
DoB:	Affix label here

Day no: _ _ _ _ _ _   **Doctor doing ward round:** _ _ _ _ _ _ _ _ _ _ _ _ _ _ _ _

Date: _ _ _ _ _ _ _ _   **Time:** _ _ _ _ _ _ _   **Admitting doctor:** _ _ _ _ _ _ _ _ _ _ _ _ _ _ _

Diagnosis	1	
	2	
	3	
	4	
	5	

Airway *Please tick*	Own	CEOTT	Trache	Day *Record number*

Breathing *Please tick/complete boxes where applicable*

Spontaneous ventilation	T piece	Facemask		Fi0$_2$
CPAP	Pressure			
BiPAP	PEEP high	PEEP low		

Ventilator mode

	PS	PC	PEEP	pH
	Set Rate		Peak Paw	P$_a$C0$_2$
	V$_T$	V$_E$	I:E ratio	HC0$_3$ / P$_a$0$_2$
RR				B/E
ETC0$_2$				Sa0$_2$
SpC0$_2$				Hb
Secretions:			Resp. drugs:	
CXR:				

Circulation			Inotropes:	µg/kg/min
Cap. refill		secs		µg/kg/min
HR	(MAP)			µg/kg/min
BP	CVP	cm H$_2$0		µg/kg/min
HS	Rhythm		Other drugs:	
Art.line: site		Day		
CVP line: site		Day		

Disability/Neurology			
Pupils R		GCS; E	/ 4
L		M / 6 =	/ 15
A V P U (please circle)		V / 5	
Sedation	mg/hr		mg/hr
Analgesia			
Observations			
Renal		**Abdo**	
Balance last 24hrs	mls	Nutrition:	
U/O range last 24hrs	ml/hr	TPN? Y/N If yes, mls/hr	
Diuretics:		NG? Y/N If yes, mls/hr	
		Oral? Y/N	
		Bowels open Y/N	
Urea Sodium		BM Insulin s/s u/hr	
Creatinine Potassium			
Drains: Site: Vol last 24hrs		Site: Vol last 24hrs	
Micro/sepsis			
Core temp °C		Antibiotics: Day	
WCC CRP		Day	
Antibiotic levels		Day	
		Day	
PT: INR: APTT:		Plt: Anticoagulated: Y/N	
Ortho/trauma		**Other drugs**	
C spine immobilised Y/N		Fractures	
Other			
Problems		**Plan**	
		Signed _	

VARIATION RECORD

Ward: _ _ _ _ _ _ _ _ _ _ _ _ _ _

Date: _ _ _ _ _ _ _ _ _ _ _ _ _ _

Name:	Hospital no:
DoB:	Affix label here

Profession; D=doctor, N=Nurse, OT=Occupational therapist, DT=Dietitian, PH=Physiotherapist, SW=Social worker, SLT=Speech and language therapist, SPEC=Specialist nurse

Date and time	Profession (enter code)	Variation report	Signature

HOURLY RECORD OF CARE

Ward: **ITU**	Hosp no:	Name:	DoB:

Date: Time																				
Respiratory system (see GPP)																				
Hourly observations carried out																				
Patient is breathing spontaneously																				
F1O2 > 50%																				
CPAP																				
BIPAP																				
IPPV																				
ETT																				
Tracheostomy present?																				
ETT or tracheostomy suction performed																				
Respiratory arrest?																				
Cardiovascular system																				
Hourly observations carried out																				
Cardiac monitoring																				
Inatropes																				
Arterial line in use (see care guide)																				
CVP line in situ																				
CVP measurements taken																				
IV access – no. of cannulae																				
Cannula 1 – phlebitis score is 0																				
Record site if it changes																				
Cannula 2 – phlebitis score is 0																				
Record site if it changes																				
Cannula 3 – phlebitis score is 0																				
Record site if it changes																				
Cannula 4 – phlebitis score is 0																				
Record site if it changes																				
Blood / blood products transfused																				
Clotting disorder present?																				
Cardiac arrest?																				
Gastro-intestinal system																				
NG tube in situ																				
J tube in situ																				
Enteral feeding as prescribed																				
TPN as prescribed																				
Patient has vomited																				
Bowels opened																				

Please indicate care given/observations carried out by: Y = yes   N = no   Continue overleaf

Please write variations from routine care on the variation record

Date:	Time													
Genito-urinary system														
Urine measured hourly														
IV replacement is = or > 1–4 hourly														
Electrolytes have been monitored														
Clotting disorder present?														
Paracentesis (see care guide)														
Central nervous system														
Neurological observations carried out														
Sedatives given since last assessment														
Mobility risk assessment up to date														
Pain														
Epidural as prescribed														
PCA as prescribed														
PRN analgesia given														
Other care														
Surgical wound care guide has been followed														
Surgical drain care guide has been followed														
Patient feels clean and comfortable														
Mouthcare care guide has been followed														
Patient has had a shave														
Patient has had a hair wash														
MRSA swabs taken?														
MRSA care guide followed														
Other care guides used (list below)														
Complex care plans in use (list below)														
To be signed by the nurse who carries out each assessment/recording of care given														

Please write variations from routine care on the variation record.

Glossary of terms

Caldicott
Review led by Dame Fiona Caldicott into the use of patient-identifiable information for non-clinical purposes with recommendations on appropriate safeguards to govern access to and storage of such information.

Clinical governance
A national framework through which NHS organisations are accountable for continuously improving the quality and clinical effectiveness of their services.

Clinical terms
Clinical terms are concepts embedded in a thesaurus that enables healthcare professionals to select terms for use in an electronic health record. Concepts are embedded within a hierarchy that provides the user with a means of navigating through search procedures. Synonyms for specific concepts are provided within the framework that allow the user to use different routes for selecting terms, e.g. cancer/carcinoma. Clinical terms (i.e. SNOMED RT) should allow the full integration of all medical information in the electronic patient record into a single data structure, facilitating interoperability between a wide variety of systems and medical records.

Clinicians
Those directly involved in the care and treatment of patients, including doctors, dentists, nurses, midwives, health visitors, pharmacists, opticians, orthoptists, chiropodists, radiographers, physiotherapists, dietitians, occupational therapists, medical laboratory scientific officers, orthotists

and prosthetists, therapists, speech and language therapists, and all other healthcare professionals.

Electronic health record (EHR)
The term EHR is used to describe the concept of a longitudinal record of patients' health and healthcare – cradle to grave. It combines both the information about patient contacts with primary healthcare as well as subsets of information associated with the episodic elements of care held in EPRs.

Electronic patient record (EPR)
A record containing a patient's personal details (name, date of birth, etc.), their diagnosis or condition and details about the treatment/assessments undertaken by a clinician. Typically covers the episodic care provided mainly by one institution.

Health professionals
See Clinicians.

ICP
An integrated care pathway determines locally agreed, multidisciplinary practice based on guidelines and evidence where available, for a specific patient/client group. It forms all or part of the clinical record, documents the care given and facilitates the evaluation of outcomes for continuous monitoring.

Multidisciplinary team
A combination of professionals who contribute to patient care, including doctor, nurse, physiotherapist, occupational therapist, social worker, specialist nurse, ward clerk, secretary, coder, healthcare assistant, auxiliary nurse, volunteer.

National Clinical Information Programme
National initiative to coordinate and develop work on clinical information, including Codes, Terms, Headings, Messaging, Clinical Record Management, Education and Professional Development, Data Quality and the Security and Confidentiality Advisory Group.

National Institute for Clinical Excellence (NICE)
A Special Health Authority established to promote clinical best practice.

National Service Frameworks
Models of how services should be provided, in order to improve the quality of patient care and to address unacceptable variations in services

across the country. NSFs are a key part of the NHS quality initiatives, covering all areas of service delivery. This covers setting national standards and defining service models for a specific service or care group, programmes to support implementation, establishing performance measures against which progress within an agreed timescale will be measured.

NHS Direct
Nurse-led telephone service to the public, currently being piloted, providing advice on health and health services.

NHS Information Authority (NHSIA)
The Special Health Authority that leads the implementation of *Information for Health.*

NHSnet
A communications network designed to support electronic communications between NHS users quickly and securely.

NHS Number
A unique number that identifies a patient. Everyone will be allocated a number.

NHS Strategic Tracing Service
Service provided to NHS organisations to enable them to obtain an NHS Number for individual patients.

NHS trusts
Statutory public bodies providing NHS hospital and community healthcare.

OPCS-4
Coding system used to record procedures carried out during delivery of healthcare.

Outcome indicators
Measurements of the success of clinical treatment/intervention in terms of the impact on the health of the individual.

Primary care
Family health services provided by a range of practitioners, including family doctors (GPs), community nurses, dentists, pharmacists, optometrists and ophthalmic medical practitioners.

Secondary care
Specialist care, typically provided in a hospital setting or following referral from a primary or community health professional.

SNOMED
SNOMED is the Systematised Nomenclature of Human and Veterinary Medicine. It is a comprehensive, multiaxial nomenclature classification work created for the indexing of the entire medical record, including signs and symptoms, diagnoses and procedures.

Telemedicine/Telecare
Any healthcare related activity (including diagnosis, advice, treatment and monitoring) that normally involves a professional and a patient (or one professional and another) who are separated in space (and possibly also in time) and is facilitated through the use of information and communications technologies. Telemedicine is usually delivered in a hospital clinic or surgery, while telecare is delivered in the patient's home.

White Papers
The New NHS: modern, dependable, Command Paper 3807, published in December 1997. Sets out the government's programme for the modernisation of the NHS.

Further reading

- Aggleton P and Chalmers A (2000) *Nursing Models and Nursing Practice* (2e). Macmillan Press, London.
- Audit Commission (1997) *Setting the Records Straight*. Audit Commission, London.
- Caine C and Kendrick M (1997) The role of clinical directorate managers in facilitating evidence-based practice: a report of an exploratory study. *J Nurs Manag.* **5**(3): 157–65.
- Cotter A (2001) Improving services for older people. *Prof Nurse.* **16**(5): 11–32.
- Currell R, Wainwright P and Urquart C (2000) *Nursing Record Systems: effects on nursing practice and healthcare outcomes* (Cochrane Review). The Cochrane Library, Issue 4. Update Software, Oxford.
- Currell R, Gold G, Hardiker N *et al.* (1998) *The Nursing Information Research Project. Final report for the project board*. NHS Centre for Coding and Classification. The NOMINA Group, Leicester.
- Department of Health (1997) *The New NHS: modern, dependable*. HMSO, London.
- Department of Health (2001) *Building the Information Core: implementing The NHS Plan*. HMSO, London.
- Department of Health (2001) *The Essence of Care: patient-focused benchmarking for healthcare practitioners*. DoH, London. www.doh.gov.uk/essenceofcare
- Gift AG (1989) Visual analogue scales: measurement of subjective phenomena. *Nurs Res.* **38**(5): 286–8.
- Kennedy C and Arundel D (1998) District nurses' knowledge and practice of wound assessment. *Br J Nurs.* **7**(8): 481–6.
- King's Fund (1997) *Turning Evidence into Everyday Practice*. King's Fund, London.
- Kneale J (2000) Evidence-based practice and orthopaedic nursing. *J Orthopaed Nurs.* **4**(1): 16–21.
- Lorenzi NM and Riley RT (1994) *Organisational Aspects of Health Informatics: managing technological change*. Springer-Verlag, New York.

- Lorenzi NM and Riley RT (2000) Managing change: an overview. *J Am Med Inform Assoc.* **7**: 116–24.
- Lorig K (1984) Measurement of pain. *Nurs Res.* **33**: 376.
- Lowe C (1998) Care pathways: have they a place in 'the new National Health Service'? *J Nurs Manag.* **6**: 303–6.
- Mackintosh IP (2001) *Information for Health Local Implementation Strategy.* Avon IM&T Consortium, Bristol.
- Manley K (2000) Organisational culture and consultant nurse outcomes. *Nurs Crit Care.* **5**(4): 179–86.
- Middleton S and Roberts A (1998) *Clinical Pathways Workbook.* VFM, Wales.
- Morison B and Baker C (2001) Tissue viability: how to raise the awareness of pressure sore prevention. *Br J Midwif.* **9**(3): 147–50.
- Naylor CD (2001) Clinical decisions: from art to science and back again. *Lancet.* **358**: 523–4.
- NHS Executive (2000) *The NHS Plan.* NHSE, London.
- NHS Executive Information Policy Unit (1998) *Working Together with Health Information: a partnership strategy for education, training and development.* Department of Health, London.
- NHS Executive Information Policy Unit (2000) *Working in Partnership: developing a whole systems approach.* Department of Health, London.
- NHS Information Authority (1999) *Information for Practice: the national information management agenda and you.* NHSIA, London. www.nhsia.nhs.uk/nhid/pages/resource_informatics/default.asp
- NHS Information Authority (1999) *Towards an Information Standard for Organising Clinical Communications: a position paper.* Department of Health, London.
- Page S and Meerabeau L (2000) Achieving change through reflective practice: closing the loop. *Nurse Educ Today.* **20**(5): 365–72.
- Polit D and Hungler B (1999) *Nursing Research Principles and Methods* (6e). Lippincott, Philadelphia, PA.
- Severs M and Pearson C (1999) *Learning to Manage Health Information: a theme for clinical education.* Enabling People Programme, Bristol. NHS Executive, London.
- Suderman EM, Deatrich JV, Johnson LS and Sawatsky-Dickson DM (2000) Action research sets the stage to improve discharge preparation. *Paed Nurs.* **26**(6): 571–6, 583–4.
- Underwood F and Parker J (1998) Developing and evaluating an acute stroke care pathway through action research. *Nurse Res.* **6**(2): 27–38.
- Wewers ME and Lowe NK (1990) A critical review of visual analogue scales in the measurement of subjective phenomena. *Res Nurs Health.* **13**: 227–36.
- Volmink J, Swingler G and Seigfried N (2001) Where to practice evidence-based medicine? *Lancet.* **357**: 723–4.

Index